"Well...
What Did the Doctor Say?"

Stories From the Bedside
by
James V. Ferguson, M.D.

Also by James V. Ferguson, MD
Epiphany, a novel

ISBN #978-1-4951-5074-6

Introduction

I've been teaching patients and offering advice for forty years. My wife often quips that you should be careful when asking my opinion; you may get it even if you didn't ask. However, being a physician and offering medical advice has been my life's work.

Three things caused me to consider this book. The first can be blamed on Charles Krauthammer, the celebrated writer and thinker, who recently published a memorable collection of his essays. The second is the changing medical climate in America which compelled me to leave my large traditional medical practice for a small concierge practice. The emphasis on the bottom line and herd management rather than the individual patient drove me away and afforded me time to compile these essays from my newspaper column in the Knoxville Focus.

*The third and real reason for this collection is told in the first essay, **The Christmas Gift**. You should at least take time to read this story even if you don't buy my book. Other essays deal with medicine, science, spirituality, history, politics, art, philosophy and even travel, all told within the context of my internal medicine practice.*

I hope you'll enjoy these stories as much as I did crafting them. It has been interesting rereading my essays and recalling the lives of patients. Many have asked me where my stories come from. My response has always been, "They walk into my office, usually with a medical problem, and that's where the story begins."

I want to say, "Thank you!" to my patients for all the stories, but most of all the relationships. And I need to thank my wife Becky, my "editress," and my life-partner who always thinks the best of me whether I deserve it or not. And lastly, a special thank you goes to Mrs. C whose story must be first.

TABLE OF CONTENTS

The Christmas Gift - January 6, 2014

Several years ago I wrote an essay that referred to a short story by O. Henry called **The Gift of the Magi**. If you've never read this gem, you must. It is a story of the perfect Christmas gift that is born of love and respect. The title alludes to the visit of the Magi at Epiphany celebrated each year, twelve days after Christmas.

Some people complain that Christmas has become too commercial, and that it's hard to find a special gift in a country where most of us have all we need. As my readers know, I love Christmas movies, and often count on them to get me in the Holiday spirit. **National Lampoon's Christmas Vacation** is a staple for me and my son-in-law Ryand. You may remember one scene where Clark Griswold (played by Chevy Chase) receives a membership in the jelly-of-the-month club. He was not amused when his cousin Eddie tells him that this gift is one that "keeps on giving."

We've all gotten Christmas gifts that – shall we say – did not strike a chord. However, this year I received the greatest Christmas gift since Santa brought me a bazooka when I was eight years old. Mrs. C has been my patient for a long time and not infrequently would comment on my weekly newspaper essays during her office visits. In fact, she's told me more than once she's collected every story I've ever written for the Focus. I guess you could say I was flattered, but I was – as the British say – gobslapped when she made an appointment with me late in December, 2013 to say goodbye and to bring my Christmas gift.

I "remember" my doctors at Christmas usually with a gift card to a restaurant, a bottle of wine or some of my wife Becky's homemade treats. The saying goes "it's not the gift, but the thought that counts." This year Ms. C caused me to pause and reflect on not only O. Henry's short story, but the lesson of the widow's mite told in the Gospels of Mark and Luke. In this story a poor widow gives lovingly and sacrificially. Ms. C is soon to enter the hospital for serious surgery, but before her ordeal she gave me her collection of all my essays bound in three volumes. I am rarely speechless, but on December 23rd, 2013, at 2:32 PM, I was.

Writers seldom go back and read their work. Perhaps it's because they find too many errors or poor sentences or things they wish they had said better. Ms. C's gift may change that perspective for me and cause me to publish a book of my essays. I told her (and others like her) that she was the reason I've continued so long in our broken medical system. I take care of some patients out of duty and professionalism. Others I love and enjoy. I told her I would not miss some in the former group, but she would not be among those.

This holiday season was like no other for me. I graduated from medical school in

1975, and doctors of my era went into practice assuming patients would sometimes become ill at night or on holidays. Dragging out of bed and to the hospital at 2 AM is not fun, but this went with the title M.D. Things are different now, and I've come to accept the changes, though I don't agree the changes are best for patients. Ms. C's visit on the 23rd was my last day in my medical practice. My last night on call was Christmas Eve. And then as the ball dropped in Times Square my career in traditional medicine was over.

Change is inevitable and is reflected in New Year's Resolutions which I never used to make. As I think back over the years I sense that I was always going somewhere. In college I studied hard to get into medical school. In medical school I worked to acquire the foundational education of my profession. A postdoctoral residency program in internal medicine was my next challenge, and then I worked to build a practice and raise a family. My daughter, Jenny, recently asked me how I was doing with all the changes in my life. I shared with her my perceptional journey. As she mucked horse stalls on our mini farm, she told me that I had "arrived." And as my grandson Oakley sped by us on his Christmas wagon I knew she was right. I have arrived because I have no more mountains to climb and I'm where I need and want to be.

I once read that the most important job you'll ever have is raising a child. I believe this is true, but for most of my adult life I found that everything was done around my days on call and my office medical practice. My kids were fortunate that they had two parents with divided but overlapping duties. I worked and supported the family financially. Becky managed our home and nurtured our kids. In all of human history this is the ways things have been. I believe it could have been the other way around, but Becky's nurturing skills are superior to mine and it worked well for our family.

I'm told this is antiquated thinking and that I need to change my perspective. I believe I'll side with the lessons of history and my principles instead of the philosophy of "modern liberalism." After all, how's that working?

The Gift of the "Fer-Guy" - January 4, 2010

"How long ye in for?" I asked the man next to me as I dropped into a chair beside him, strategically placed for men Christmas shopping with their wives.

"Oh, I've got about another hour on my sentence," he sighed deeply. I responded with a knowing nod that all men understand. It has been one of my observations that women shop and men buy. There are, of course, exceptions to this rule, but Becky acknowledges that even if she were to find the perfect gift for a great price she'd need to confirm this by looking at all the alternatives. Men and women are different.

My new friend pointed at the bags scattered all around my feet and said, "We ain't much more than a couple of pack mules, are we?"

I laughed at his tongue-in-cheek humor, enjoying the male bonding common among *pack mules*. I didn't tell him that I'd volunteered to come Christmas shopping with my wife, feeling a bit guilty that she usually does the bulk of our shopping. I do help around the house and in other ways, but mostly it's Becky who makes our house a home.

Actually, I was on a mission the Saturday before Christmas. I had been actively listening to my wife for Christmas suggestions over the last two and a half months. As Christmas approached I became more desperate and resorted to asking her directly for suggestions, only to hear that she "didn't need anything." It's true that Becky and I are blessed and want for little of substance. But it's Christmas, for Heaven's sake, and I've got to have something for her on Christmas morning besides stocking stuffers entrusted to "Santa". I even began asking my patients for suggestions. The best suggestion came from a lady who said to "give her something from the heart."

One of my favorite stories is **The Gift of the Magi** by O. Henry. This short story about a young couple at Christmas can be found with a simple Google search and then savored. The gifts of Dell and Jim exemplify the Spirit of Christmas and the sacrificial giving that the Greeks referred to as agape.

I can't say that my gift compares to the Wise Men's gifts at Epiphany two thousand years ago; nor can I say that I gave sacrificially as the couple in O. Henry's story. But, I think I did pretty well – even for a guy.

Many years ago we were troubled with a series of break-ins at our home. One time the thieves even went through my wife's jewelry and took *nothing*. That insult has **cost** me plenty over the years and I did penance and vowed never to be the victim of such scorn again!

You might ask what this vignette has to do with medicine. I might reply that this story is about relationships, commitment and love for the person that you share your life with. We've all heard it said that "if momma ain't happy, ain't nobody gonna be happy." But it goes far beyond this. Thirty-four years ago I chose a partner for life, and I believe that this contract is renegotiated everyday by working on my marriage. If you think you can neglect your partner, your family, or your spiritual relationship and assume they won't wither, then you need to talk with your doctor, counselor, and minister. How's that for a New Year's resolution?

So you see being with your wife shopping, even if only hauling bags around for her, is relationship building. Sending cards, writing personal emails, or connecting with loved ones by phone is relationship building.

I've heard it said that if you love something you spend time with *her*. But a special Christmas frill helps if you're really desperate!

I love double entendres. And I love finding the perfect word or phrase to capture the moment or convey the thought. I wasn't always that way. In fact I was an underachiever until I went to college and buckled down. I've changed a lot since I came of age, and I think I know where the journey from "the far country" began.

As I look back I can tell people with certainly that I was a fool until my mid-twenties. Yes, I had a lot of facts in my head which I eventually organized into a compendium of useful knowledge. But somewhere along the way I acquired a modicum of wisdom. Perhaps this originated from a passion for learning things just for the sheer joy of knowing. I don't know where this desire came from, but I can identify with Star Trek's Mr. Spock who often exclaims, "Fascinating!"

The ancient Greeks called the passionate quest for understanding "gnosis", from which the word knowledge comes to us. My patient Mr. T has knowledge that I don't possess. As we discuss his medical issues we often chit-chat about family, jobs and our life's journey. Mr. T is a great gardener and though farming is not his vocation it is his passion. I'm blessed to be counted as his neighbor and friend, with whom he shares his bounty. I told him about my project to improve our property and my plans for a big garden this year. And that's when my education began.

"Trying to plow *new ground* with a tiller won't work, Doc. Ya gotta bust up that sod with a plow." He was right of course. I'd been killing myself using a gasoline driven tiller. I can only imagine what it must have been like to fell trees with an ax, then pull the stumps by mule or ox, and then break up the ground to make it ready for seeds using only a spade or an antiquated plow. You may be interested to learn that the modern plow was only invented about 200 years ago and George Washington was using technology that was little different from the Romans. We've certainly "come a long baby" since John Deere invented his "plow" in 1837.

A colleague once challenged me that my passion for the care of my patients can only go so far. She said, "You can't care more than they do, Jim." What a profound observation which I've *chewed on* many times since then. How much can a doctor do to make a difference in someone's life and health? I suspect that I've rubbed some patients wrong as I ask them again how they're doing with their smoking. If I put myself in a smoker's shoes I can imagine that being asked repeatedly is analogous to having one's shortcomings pointed out again and again. If it wasn't so important to the health of my folks, I'd give it a rest. Objective data shows that smoking cessation is more important than controlling blood pressure, treating diabetes, and certainly more beneficial than lowering someone's cholesterol with medications.

A patient once asked me if I'd ever smoked. I hedged saying, "I'll bet that smoking grape vines in Boy Scout outings doesn't count." I then told him that when I completed my internal medicine residency my colleagues and I had a big party and we drank some beer that night. I confessed that someone took a picture of me smoking a cigar, but I have no recollection of it.

In the Gospel of Luke the Master is recorded telling a story about a sower of seeds. The metaphor of seeds falling on hardpan resonates with me and anyone else who has tried to throw grass seed on bare spots in the yard without first tilling the soil. I've observed this enterprise to be quite fruitless. Similarly, our receptiveness to medical advice or Spiritual nudging can only occur when new ground is made ready for the seeds of a better way.

As I drive into work each morning I think about the day before me and its challenges. I think about the people I will see and the seeds that I'll plant in hopefully fallow soil. For some time now my mantra has been to ask for strength and courage to speak the truth in a loving and caring way. And my goal is to do my best, to do my duty for God and country and those that I serve.

At the end of the day I know when I've been successful and when I could have done better. It's then that I fall back on the words of the Master who said, "Grace is sufficient." With this blessed assurance I can go on tilling the soil 'til the "race is finished."

"As you do unto the least of these you do unto me."
Matthew 25:40

It was pitch black and raining sideways as we made our way up the muddy road to make the house call. I do house calls less often now, but Diva is a special lady.

Becky accompanied me on this mission, not because she has special medical training, but because it takes two people to do Diva's treatments. My wife is a wonderful person and most creatures sense her goodness. I was counting on her ability to entertain Ms. Diva so the "doctor" could apply his talents.

Thankfully, we were able to drive right into the barn where our patient greeted us with an extended head through the window of her stall. You see, Diva is my daughter's horse who has a severe eye injury and we were there for the late night antibiotic drops administered through a tunneled catheter under her eyelid. Diva doesn't understand that we're trying to save her eye. She's an 1100 pound filly with the brain of a *one year old* and an attitude befitting her name. Fortunately, she does understand apples and carrots and peppermint candies, so our mission was ultimately successful that night.

My family loves animals and we've had a lot of experience with the University of Tennessee Veterinary Hospital. It's really a blessing to have this center of veterinary excellence in our Knoxville community. We hear a lot these days about the expense of medical care, but when your loved one or your beloved pet is sick most of us do what is necessary. Perhaps even the disgraced football player Michael Vick has acquired some new empathy from the time spent in his prison cell. I'm told the Master does some of His best work in prison cells and hospital beds.

It's now Wednesday and we return to the Vet Hospital to see Dr. Ward, Diva's ophthalmologist, and his compassionate staff. His *exam room* is understandably larger than mine and has a sloping floor for easy cleaning. Thankfully, most of my patients are "potty trained" and continent. The exam room's only adornments are horse pictures on his computer's screen saver.

Taking a horse to the doctor is no small issue. It requires manpower and expertise to maneuver a large skittish patient into a trailer and chauffeur her across town. The logistics are somewhat akin to an ambulance ride with an EMT crew, only tougher.

As I watched Dr. Ward examine Diva's wounded eye, I asked the doctors and staff how an animal as fragile as a horse can be explained by Darwin's theory of evolutionary survival of the fittest. A senior physician hesitated and then said, "That's a very interesting question; I don't know the answer."

I told him, no matter; my mind just wants to know the why of things. Philosophically, internists start from a science based perspective and the theory of *why* things occur. The *why* then determines *what* is wrong and can be done about it. Life is complicated and every patient is unique and different. I've spoken about medical care guidelines in previous essays and how protocols can work in situations that are straightforward, but they are woefully inadequate when something out of the ordinary occurs.

The University of Tennessee Vet School has all the medical specialties, including internists like me who also ask "Why?" I spoke to several regarding the evolution of horses and the conclusion is that horses in the wild are probably hardier than our domesticated and highly bred *Divas*. The experts posited that wild horses wouldn't survive to reproduce unless they were tough. Perhaps it's good to be a mongrel with genetic diversity rather than a thoroughbred. Inbreeding can produce genius or disaster and is therefore proscribed by laws promulgated in the Middle Ages. Perhaps we Americans have "bred" dependency into our people with disastrous results.

As I reflect on the coming winter, I wonder if I'd be strong enough or resourceful enough to survive without all the civilization around me. "Homo sapiens" means wise man. Evolution theory says that we *wise* men came from ancestors who no longer exist. Our survival advantage is our intelligence. So far we've been a very successful species.

I believe our country is likewise exceptional. I hope it's hardy enough to survive the tough times that are coming. Some think America's been successful because God chose us. I like my wife Becky's perspective better. She believes that America's been successful because we chose God.

Let's not forget this **reason for the season**.

One of my favorite paintings is *The Doctor* by Sir Luke Fildes. Painted in 1887, it hangs in London's Tate Museum, and depicts a doctor making a house-call on a sick child. The painting is a study in contrasts: a tilted lamp shade casts light on the tiny patient stretched between two chairs as the worried father looks on from the darkness in the back of the room; the doctor is a study in concentration like Rodin's epic sculpture *The Thinker*, while the child's mother collapses in tears. I studied the painting closely looking for the doctor's bag, but unfortunately for this child the proverbial bag of tricks was nowhere to be seen.

You can easily find and view this most famous of medical paintings on the internet. I've always loved the covers of *The Journal of the American Medical Association* (JAMA) which depicts great art that is then explained by JAMA's resident art critic. For years the keen observations of M. Therese Southgate, MD would engage me. She is now retired, but her description of Grandma Moses' colors "as fresh as new Crayolas on the first day of school" still resonates in my soul and gives me shivers of joy.

I don't want to diverge into art criticism, even though things of beauty "are a joy forever" as Keats once said. And I used to serve as a docent at the Knoxville Museum of Art. This week, my mind has been on the iconic doctor's bag as I convert to electronic medical records (EMR) and wax a bit nostalgic over the changes in my profession.

I've been preparing for this revolutionary conversion for the last nine months, but now my patients and I are living it. I'll admit I drug my feet, but the Obama-care legislation says I must submit or quit practicing medicine. The fact is I'm not ready to quit, so to escape the escalating fines, I will convert to EMR which some refer to as EHR (electronic health records).

After spending a long and final day with a personal tutor, I was declared ready for 21st century medical care with EMR. I was tired as I made rounds on my hospitalized patients that evening, but I was struck to see a colleague walking down the hall to his next patient carrying a lap top computer rather than a doctor's bag. At the nurse's station I empathized with another older colleague as he groused about electronic records which the new order was forcing upon him. He swore to me that the post-it note on the hospital's computer screen was not his doing. It read "Meaningful use [of computers] will make your hair fall out."

I'm not an EMR troglodyte as a former colleague once quipped derisively. I can see some good in this new technology, but it must never replace a caring and thinking physician, or we're lost. I refuse to exchange my stethoscope for a mouse. When I came of *medical* age in 1975, a scandalous book called *The House of God* was a rite of passage for all young doctors. The story reveals the crass observations of an intern who is taught how to make the patient's medical chart look good – "Buff the chart" was the advice then (and perhaps now with the Veteran's Administration).

We doctors must resist the siren's song of point-and-click medical data entry to make the chart look good. We must stay focused on our patients as did Sir Luke Fildes' doctor in his epic painting. We must guard against our conclusions becoming lost amidst pages of verbiage designed to satisfy Medicare's requirements of documentation that studies have shown increase doctors' charges by 40%!

Actually, the basics of medical care are pretty straight forward and are embodied in the old **SOAP** note format – the **S**ubjective story of the patient, **O**bjective findings of the doctor, his **A**ssessment or conclusions, and the **P**lan of treatment. I remember going to my family doctor as a teenager and seeing my entire medical record scribbled on 4X6 index cards. This was, of course, far superior to no record keeping with the impoverished patients we served in Guatemala on mission trips, but pales in comparison to our marvelous EMR tool which enables us to store voluminous medical data.

We do have a contingency protocol in the event of a power outage and our EMR crashes. We have an emergency kit that contains a large ring notebook describing how to use the system, and under it two note pads and #2 pencils! You can't make this kind of stuff up.

As I finish this essay, I'm glad to report that I've survived the conversion, and so have my patients. I've rearranged my exam rooms so that my patients sit beside me as I concentrate on their story and make notes with my hunt-and-peck keyboard skills. Details are later recorded with another new technology that I learned this week, the Dragon voice-recognition dictation system.

Yes, this is a *brave new world* as Miranda observed in Shakespeare's *Tempest*. And I'm sure I'll be fine, that is unless I get a cold and the Dragon system no longer recognizes my accentuated East Tennessee nasal twang.

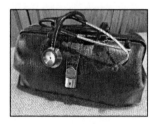

There's no accounting for taste. I don't know why I love cabbage and detest Brussels sprouts. I know I have a Southerner's taste because I love collard greens, grits and fried okra. Obviously, taste is a personal thing. Count Basie perhaps said it best observing that "if it sounds good, it is."

If you ask someone how many senses we have, most would say five and list sight, hearing, touch, smell and taste. In fact, our brain sits inside our skull, shielded from the light of day and is dependent on the senses to bring data to it for interpretation. The brain doesn't even feel pain because it lacks the sensory apparatus to register painful stimuli.

As an empiricist, I observe the world through my senses. I can see that the stop light is red and I can hear the music of Puccini. I enjoy my wife's soft touch, the smell of her perfume and consider her peach-berry pie sublime. All these sensations are registered on my sensory organs and then transmitted by the nervous system to my brain. It's the brain's job to sort it all out and define my reality.

Can your senses lie to you? Can your eyes deceive you? This is a relevant question with modern digital imaging and the ability to photo shop images. But even in the 17th century, Thomas Hobbs considered his senses subject to bias, and his contemporary René Descartes went so far as to isolate himself in his room where he finally concluded, "Cogito ergo sum" (I think therefore I am).

Taking empiricism to the extreme, John Barkley wondered if a tree makes a noise when it falls in the forest if there's no one there to hear it. There's a modern corollary to Barkley's conundrum that wonders if a husband is still wrong if his wife is not there to correct him.

Textbooks tell us that we humans perceive four taste sensations – sweet, sour, salty and bitter. But taste is complex and related to other senses. Try tasting something with your nose pinched or plugged with a cold. And the texture of food matters as does the visual presentation. I've observed that food tastes differently if served on china versus a paper plate. And Becky's southern sweet tea is best when served in a tall glass rather than in a Styrofoam cup.

Experience tells me there's more to this taste thing than meets the tongue. You'd probably become bored if I discussed the anatomy of the tongue and its 10,000 taste buds. Eyes might cross discussing the science of dissolved chemicals which bind to taste bud sensory receptors and generate electrochemical signals which race to the brain at 50 meters a second. Yes, this might be a bit arcane or pedantic for the Focus.

More interesting was an ad I saw recently for Kikkoman Soy Sauce that alluded to a fifth taste called **umami**. This is actually a borrowed term from Japanese and best translates as the *savoriness* of food, notably in meat, cheese and mushrooms. Equally fascinating is that science has found the chemical responsible for umami. It is monosodium glutamate (MSG), the additive in many Asian dishes and the cause of the Asian restaurant syndrome in sensitive persons.

I've read that salsa is now the most popular American condiment, surpassing even mustard and ketchup. Certain peppers used in salsa contain the chemical *capsaicin*. This is what sets your mouth on fire. Perhaps this is another taste sensation. I only wish I had known that a habanera was lurking in the salsa my friend served us. There was little solace for me to understand why my mouth was on fire – so much for empiricism and science; bring me relief!

Becky and I love to have people over for dinner. The sharing of a meal and fellowship is a time honored custom. After all the principle sacrament of the Church surrounds a meal, and though the elites of his day were horrified, Jesus reached out to the so-called *undesirables* in the sharing of a meal.

I have only one taste precaution; beware of the chili pepper. Because this devilish plant originated in the New World, Jesus didn't have to worry about the meal Martha was preparing for him. We moderns need to be more careful.

I'm a big believer in body language, and as I walked into my patient's hospital room I felt the pall. Hippocrates once said that desperate illness often requires desperate measures. It's been my observation that it often brings out the desperation in families as well.

I'm one of the few primary care doctors who still provides care for my patients in the hospital, as well as in my office. Consequently, I'm often there during a crisis and when bad news is delivered. Experts tell me that I'm old fashioned and that specialists can take care of my folks more efficiently and better than I can. They tell me that I could make more money and have more free time if I would just accept the modern paradigm (model) of medical care and turn over the care of my patients, in their hour of greatest need, to strangers.

My patient looked frail and pale as I entered his hospital room. He had lost so much weight that his temples were sunken and he seemed lost in the white sheets of his bed. Yet, as I made my way between family members to his bedside he looked up at me with immediate recognition and obvious gladness to see a friend, who just happened to be his doctor of umpteen years. His wife even gave me a relief-filled thankful hug.

Everyone shifted to provide a place for me to sit, and then I did what I so often do: I explained to them what was going on and what the specialists were thinking. My patient liked his other doctors and they had carefully explained everything to him, but he hadn't heard it from me. And this was important because we have a long history with each other; I had *street creds* with him.

My wife says I can always find three choices for any situation. She's probably right; I'm Trinitarian at heart. I think two options aren't enough and four tend to confuse people. I quickly explained the situation to everyone, the various options, and then reassured them that the planned surgery was not only appropriate but necessary. We all have *gifts differing* as Paul wrote in Romans. My ability is the synthesis of complex medical situations and "cut to the chase."

Communication is mostly non-verbal and various studies have reported that up to three-fourths of understanding doesn't come through our ears. The point is that effective communication goes beyond what I *tell* my patients.

My professional appearance, the tone and inflection of my voice, my body language as well as facial expressions of genuine empathy all contribute mightily to what my patient and his family needed to *hear*. Poor communication and unrealistic expectations breed a lack of trust and damages the doctor-patient-family relationship. Misunderstandings lead to poor care, produce anger and even lawsuits where everyone suffers.

Elizabeth Kublai Ross wrote her sentinel work on death and dying in 1969. She said that the process of dying progresses through the stages of denial, anger, bargaining, depression and eventual acceptance. I believe illness produces the same sequence, perhaps because illness humbles us, sapping our vitality and making us more dependent on others.

Illness also puts burdens on families as they watch their loved one suffer and as they are called upon to provide care during an illness. Sometimes care-giving can overwhelm even the strongest relationship and produce desperation as a component of Dr. Ross's stages.

I'm confident that my patient will prevail; and I told him so with honesty. I never lie to folks because if you do they'll never forgive you or trust you again. It will be a tough road for him and his family, but I told him this *wasn't his time*. I told him that he had life left in him, but that he was going to have to fight to survive. And I informed him he'd be seeing a lot of me in the days ahead.

Who would have thought that a firm hand shake, a group-hug and a thumbs-up as I left the room would encourage even me?

There is a philosophy in medicine that says, "Watch one, do one, teach one." I think this perspective holds true in many avenues of life. An example is showing our kids how to tie their shoes, supervising their doing it, and then turning them loose on the world to teach others to do the same. There is no credible way to tell someone how to tie their shoes; it's a technique that must be experienced to be understood. So it is with the Grand Canyon and the Colorado River.

It's been ten days since I left the River; ten days to reflect upon this wondrous adventure. I wish I could paint a word picture adequate to describe the things I experienced, but of course that is impossible. So instead, I'll try to leave you with some impressions and the impetus to go and experience God's creation. Even our photographs are woefully inadequate when compared to that "inward eye" of memory.

As I sat journaling by the River on that last Sunday morning, with the mile high canyon rim looming above me, I imagined myself in God's mighty cathedral. The lofty interiors of medieval Gothic churches were constructed to inspire people to think, "Surely the presence of God is in this place." But these pale in comparison to the Grand Canyon. Fortunately, you don't have to take a wild ride over white water rapids to experience our Grandest Canyon. However, you must experience this wonder before you "shuffle off this mortal coil."

The Colorado River and the Grand Canyon are studies in extremes. We began our odyssey below Lake Powell and, because it was not the season of summer storms, the water was a clear Norris Lake green. We were soon sweaty in the afternoon heat and a bit apprehensive as we approached our first of eighty rapids. The calmly flowing river quickly became a maelstrom of waves that came at us from all sides, dowsing us with frigid forty-seven degree water, almost comparable to the frigid water of the north Atlantic which engulfed the Titanic. And then just as quickly the fifteen-foot waves subsided, the white water became green again and left us shaking our heads in amazement and drying in the sun.

The Colorado River's average speed is nine mph, but because water is incompressible, it accelerates to twenty-two mph when it is pinched by a narrow Canyon gorge; and the ride is exhilarating and rough. In fact, one of our guides was thrown from the raft in the middle of a class eight rapid named *Hermit* (after an old mountain coot who tried to mine asbestos along the River years ago). Many of the fourteen on our raft wore gloves to hold onto the straps positioned to keep us from being thrown overboard. There was little camera work and no adult beverages as we navigated the rapids deeper into the Canyon and backwards in geologic time as seen in the rock strata dating back 1.8 billion years. The power of water is immense and it is this erosive force that has carved the one mile deep gorge of the Canyon over the last four million years. I thought about my brother Tom as we sailed. He's a trained geologist, and the exposed thirteen different and multicolored rock layers would have him salivating.

We camped on sandbars beside the river, and on the first night I remembered why I no longer go camping. A fifty-eight year old with sore hips in need of lumbar support has trouble sleeping on a cot, especially with the cacophony of snoring people around him. The doctor in me imagined that half our party needed C-pap! And then the unexpected rain came which overwhelmed our tarps. But, we dried out and set off again to swim in turquoise streams of side canyons where big horn sheep munched on green grass that flourished next to the River despite desert conditions not fifty feet from the River's edge. We learned our lesson and put up tents the next night and were prepared for the violent thunder storm that shed torrents of rain on us and sent booming thunder through the Canyon. Even the River turned muddy brown for 24 hours after that downpour, before returning to its emerald green.

This essay was obviously not about medicine, but I write about what's on my mind and heart at the moment. Perhaps my observations will whet your appetites for adventure or the scenic wonders of our country. You owe it to yourselves and your families to experience God's cathedral, his majestic creation.

The doctor-patient relationship is a sacred thing which requires periodic nurturing. It may seem obvious to many, but I had to learn that you can't treat the condition without considering the person. Approaching a patient like Sergeant Friday on Dragnet is poor medicine. If you interact with folks, they'll trust you with the truth and often the diagnosis.

"Doc, my feet are swollen," said the usually stoic Mr. Jones. And before I could ask about important details he continued, "What'll I do about 'em?"

Some people want to know the details about their problems and others just what to do about the problem. Mr. Jones falls into the latter group, but because I believe an informed patient can better participate in their medical care I got him to listen to my circulation story.

Swollen feet are a common problem. In previous columns I've discussed heart disease and heart failure as a cause of swelling (edema). There are lots of other causes of edema, including advanced kidney or liver disease, severe malnutrition or vitamin deficiencies, certain medications or allergic reactions, toxemia of pregnancy, unusual endocrine system diseases and even exotic infections. You're probably not interested in what we internists call a "differential diagnostic" list of the conditions that cause a patient's feet to swell, but you might be interested to learn that you're designed to swell.

Imagine your heart connected to a series of pipes (arteries) that get smaller and smaller and end in a mesh of tiny blood vessels smaller than hairs. Now, envision this tangle of tiny arteries connected to a mesh of tiny veins that then get larger and larger as they return blood back towards the heart and lungs. You may have once pulled up a plant in the yard and seen the myriad of tiny roots that similarly coalesce into larger and larger roots and then the plant stem itself.

Think of your heart as a pump pushing blood with oxygen and nutrients out to the tissues of your body, and then, on reaching the tiny arteries (capillaries), the life-giving cargo is emptied, much as a dump truck would empty its cargo. At the same time wastes are absorbed into the tiny vein capillaries and eventually returned to the heart for another cycle, after first discharging the wastes and picking up a fresh load of nutrients from the liver and oxygen from the lungs. You could envision the circulatory system as a loop with the heart at one side and the capillary beds at the opposite side.

Our blood vessels are not like PVC piping or copper plumbing. They are designed to allow nutrients, oxygen, carbon dioxide and waste to move back and forth across the vessel walls. Actually, there are tiny gaps between cells that line your vessels, and this facilitates the normal physiology of your body. And since your vessels are designed to leak a bit, the Creator designed a system to pick up the excess water and return it to the circulation. This collateral *gutter* system is called the lymph circulation and has the more recognizable lymph nodes as part of the system.

Mr. Jones was patient as I went through this with him, perhaps because he drives a dump truck. However, patience only goes so far. "OK, Doc, enough stories. Why are my feet swollen?"

Swelling occurs because the heart pump fails and the circulation backs up, or something blocks the vein or lymph flow, or there is too much fluid to be handled by the system generally or locally.

Have you ever been on a long car trip and taken off your shoes only to notice that your shoes felt tight when you tried to put them back on? As you sit in a car you actually bend at the waist and the knees. This can hinder or "kink" the returning venous circulation. Additionally, when you sit, there is less pumping action of the muscles to counter the effects of gravity. And if you're overweight there is a further impediment to the returning blood flow from the legs. Add to this mix certain medications that promote swelling like ibuprofen, excessive salt ingestion, or underlying medical conditions like varicose veins, and you have a recipe for swollen feet or even a condition that we doctors call *superficial phlebitis*. This latter condition is not a blood clot in the deep vein system, but stagnant flow with resulting inflammation in the superficial smaller veins that can nonetheless be painful.

"So what should I do?" said the persistent Mr. Jones. I recommend you think physiologically about your body by avoiding excessive salt; and if you're prone to edema, elevate your legs whenever possible. It's good to get up and walk around on long trips to "pump" the veins and lymph circulation. Sometimes compression hose aid in compressing swollen veins and improving circulation. And as last resort, diuretics can be used.

"Elementary, my dear Watson, er...Mr. Jones."

The chatter became louder as I approached the end of the hospital corridor. It was late Sunday afternoon of a long weekend on call and 7N was my last stop. As I pushed a cart laden with patients' records, I sighed as I neared the room with all the chatter because I imagined a room filled with family members who would want an entire redaction of *Ms. Jones'* hospital course. Weekend care is what we doctors sometimes refer to as "problem-oriented care." In other words, we try to do what the patient needs at the moment and try not to micromanage an often complicated care plan, especially when social issues are in play. These are best managed by the patient's doctor who will "be back in the morning, rested and ready to go."

I knocked on the door as I entered only to find the room empty except for one diminutive, elderly black lady who seemed engulfed by the hospital bed and white bed sheets. She didn't seem to notice me or my cart. She was totally absorbed with the supper before her, and in between bites she continued to talk, but not to me or to anyone else. As I scanned her record I noted that she was recovering from pneumonia and had a long history of dementia. She was also on psychiatric medication to manage violent behavior. As I observed her I noted that she displayed the characteristic smacking movements of her mouth associated with certain psychiatric drugs. And then it struck me, she was talking to herself as an aid to feeding herself.

"Oh, these are good mashed potatoes," she said to herself. "Now open your mouth." And her mouth magically opened as she spooned in another bite.

As I watched in fascination I recognized the routine often employed by our nursing aides to entice and help frail patients to eat. Similar efforts are common in nursing homes. I've been known to cut up meat for patients, open milk cartons, or add creamer to coffee. Sometimes unexpected efforts by a doctor can make a difference, but this little lady was so accustomed to aides helping her, it had become an imprinted behavior from years of institutionalization.

"That's good honey," she said. "Now here's some meat; open your mouth."

Dutifully she opened her mouth again to accept the meatloaf and continued her toothless chewing, all the while describing the next bite to herself as she mixed peas with the mashed potatoes.

"Oh, dem's nice peas," she said, "and here's some with mashed potatoes. Now, open your mouth," and she did it again and again without anyone to notice her routine other than me, her doctor for the day.

I've thought about this magical and bitter-sweet moment often over the years. The mood altering drugs that caused Ms. Jones' lip smacking condition (tardive dyskinesia) are not often used these days and most psychiatric institutions are long since gone. However, we still have a lot of frail and vulnerable people in *extended care facilities*, as they are now called to avoid the pejorative term of nursing homes. No one wants to be a burden to others, leave their home where they're comfortable, or go to a nursing home. In fact, any change of venue can lead to confusion and agitation in people with damaged brains or dementia.

I recently saw one of my 95-year-old patients at a skilled nursing home where she was convalescing and receiving therapy for a severely fractured ankle. The facility was clean, the staff was friendly, there was no smell, and my patient even praised the food. No, she is not demented! The point is, we sometimes have to do what is necessary and there are many options of care ranging from community assisted living to what we still refer to as nursing home care. The emphasis is *care*.

In the future I hope more care will be delivered at home by people trained to provide this service. Our locally based **College of Direct Support** offers this training. And medical organizations such as the ACP and even the government and insurance companies are recognizing the advantages of home-based care managed by a doctor. They refer to this **new program** as the *Patient Centered Medical Home.* Imagine that!

Lately, I've been spending a lot of time in hospital waiting rooms. The first circumstance was during my daughter's labor and delivery; that was a blessing. This time it's not fun, but ominous, so now I wait with my family for the results of surgery and hopefully the doctor's reassurance that the enlarging tumor is not cancer.

I'm familiar with waiting rooms where families wait to hear word of their loved ones. I often think about those poor people who wait for hours for scraps of information or solace. I often see them from the corner as I walk by the intensive care unit (ICU) on my hospital rounds. Updates on a patient's condition are so necessary and helpful even if things aren't going well. This aspect of medicine is the art of caring and we doctors must never forget this vital lesson.

Doctors have to be careful about the words they use and remember everyone hears something different. I'm keenly aware that sometimes what a patient or a family understands is different from what I've said. I like to identify a spokesperson when I speak with a family in the ICU. I'm especially careful in the emotionally charged situation of illness that can color people's perception. That's a recipe for adding to a family's anguish or engendering mistrust.

As we wait for my daughter's surgeon, I think about how I feel to be on **the other side**. Maybe there's a further lesson in empathy for me. Because I'm the doctor in our extended family, I'm frequently asked medical questions. What might I do or say in this situation? I realize that my role is to just be here and to offer up prayers. I realize that I'm powerless to directly help the surgeon or even the pathologist who will decide if the tumor is cancerous. Becky is an expert on this side of medicine, and firmly believes in the waiting room vigil. We circle the wagons during crisis even though we no longer defend against hostiles on the prairie. And we draw strength from the loved ones who wait in limbo with us.

I choose the perspective that there is purpose and plan to life. I believe this perspective is more likely than events being just subject to chance or serendipity. I often counsel patients that medical decisions are best made on **probability** rather than some remote **possibility**. We can't do CT scans on every ache and pain. You have to use common sense and consider the likelihood of serious disease.

As I sit here I wonder why bad things happen to good people. This has long been a question for humans and actually was the title of a book written by Rabbi Kushner as he pondered why his son was stricken with an incurable illness. Perhaps the apparent randomness in the universe is due to our limited vision. We moderns understand more about our world than those in past ages, but I believe there will always be some uncertainties and mysteries. And just because we don't understand something doesn't make it the result of happenstance.

I'll admit that I can't see an obvious benefit in suffering or cancer or heart attacks. Does illness occur because God doesn't care, or because of our poor choices, or because of genetics or because we've chosen our way over The Way? I don't have the answers, nor did Job or innumerable other sages over the ages. We humans have limits and I'm feeling mine as I sit here and wonder about the future and consider the feelings of others who sit in this worry-filled room.

I've been thinking a lot about prayer lately. I know that this is a medical column, but you must know by now that there's more to me than medicine. Once I was only a scientist and a rationalist. Now I embrace a spiritual perspective as well. I once thought that there was an explanation for everything. Now I see further with spiritual eyes.

We have great news! The operation is over and the surgeon tells us the tumor is benign. Life can go on, and so can I without a broken heart. There are those who would demand proof if I were to that say that my prayers were answered today. I've heard it said that there are no atheists in foxholes. Perhaps a survey should be taken in surgical waiting rooms.

I'll admit that I too often rely on my own abilities. However, when I'm in one of those "foxholes" of life I pray for courage, wisdom, and peace. And in these last few days I prayed like a child for the tumor to not be cancerous. One could argue that my surrender to competent surgeons and greater powers was rewarded with a good outcome.

Some might say that my faith perspective is nothing but a sop for my soul. Well, so what? The famous American psychologist and philosopher William James is known as the father of pragmatism, though he despised the moniker. James said in his work *The Varieties of Religious Experience* that if there are two diverse perspectives and there is no incontrovertible evidence that either is wrong, the rational man is free to choose which ever perspective works best for him.

Well said, professor. I'll choose The Way because "it makes life better now, and there is the hope of then."

I've heard it said that in retirement you work even harder. I'm not convinced of this yet, but it is different. As my readers know, I've left my traditional medical practice and I'm developing a small concierge medical practice. I guess you could say that I'm semi-retired from medicine.

Leaving my practice was a huge decision for me. When my partners and I founded our extended medical group it was a big deal in Knoxville. I've often thought about the founding of our country where the signers of The Declaration of Independence pledged, "our Lives, our Fortunes, and our Sacred Honor." In fact, Benjamin Franklin told those fifty-six signers "we must all hang together, or assuredly we shall all hang separately." My signature on our founding documents wasn't as *large* as John Hancock's, nor as risky because many of the Founders and signatories of The Declaration of Independence lost family, fortunes and some lost their lives.

I've come to conclude that I'm not retired from medicine; I'm on sabbatical like a university Don. Perhaps if doctors were able to periodically step back from their practices they might be able to return with renewed vigor. Unfortunately, in my profession you either do it 110% or not at all, unless you take the attitude of not caring, and that was impossible for me.

I'm actually catching up on my medical journals now, between walks with my grandson Oakley and chores on our mini-farm. There's less intellectual stimulation watering and feeding horses or cleaning stalls during the Polar Vortex, the media's latest example of global warming. Yes, you read that correctly. The noted scientist Al Sharpton recently explained how this cold snap is all due to man-made carbon emissions and anthropogenic global warming. Perhaps Sharpton's lunacy stems from the moniker "Al" as in Al-Gore. Perhaps the "Als" did not read the opinions of Time Magazine experts in the 1970s. The "Polar Vortex" then was said to be due to global cooling. My step-grandson, Noah asked why people believe that our record low temperatures are caused by global warming. I explained that they call it climate change now to help us overcome what our eyes tell us.

The world is certainly different now than when I first began reading medical journals. When I was on the teaching faculty of University Hospital, I often challenged medical residents with the notion, "questions never change, just the answers." I remember one resident titling his head quizzically much like a dog does when trying to triangulate the source of a sound. I told him to ponder the quote and the meaning will come to him.

Two medical articles recently caught my eye. The first appeared in the American Journal of Medicine as an editorial overview of medical genomic technology. The goal of the Human Genome Project was to define the full complement of human DNA (deoxyribonucleic acid). Each of us has a unique combination of DNA, though humans have much in common. The hope is that someday we can compare an individual's DNA against the standard human genome and make predictions about disease or even modify an aberrant area of DNA (genes) correcting a defect to effect a cure. Though tremendous progress has been made, we are not there yet.

The editorialist Dr. Joseph Alpert discussed the topic of epigenetics, or the external factors that modify or influence our DNA. He and others have postulated that our DNA is the **nature** side of the human equation. Could the **nurture** component of the equation be explained by environmental influences acting on our DNA to produce our uniqueness? Alpert describes a paper by Scherrer, et al who found vascular dysfunction in children conceived by in vitro fertilization. The thought is that the cell culture medium of these test tube babies perhaps influenced their DNA producing the measurable vascular anomalies.

A second paper in the New England Journal of Medicine summarized the mechanisms of Alzheimer's disease a complicated problem with molecular and genetic mechanisms. In 1901, Dr. Alois Alzheimer described the original case of "pre-senile dementia" in a fifty-year-old man. Dementia was not supposed to occur prior to the "expected" age of senility!

We now know that this autosomal dominant form of Alzheimer's disease is uncommon, and is thought to occur from defects in one of three genes which result in the overproduction or aggregation of the B-amyloid protein. The more common sporadic form of Alzheimer's disease is thought to result from decreased clearance of the B-amyloid protein, possibly due to genetic variation in apolipoprotein E. This fat transportation protein enables lipids (fats) to circulate in our salt water blood stream. Remember, oil and water don't mix, but proteins will dissolve in water and are thus able to transport their attached lipid molecules through the body.

Humans have three varieties of the E protein (2, 3, and 4). APO E3 is most common and confers a standard risk for dementia. E2 is actually protective of the brain; but the E4 variety is associated with Alzheimer's disease, but no one knows for sure why.

We humans still have a lot to learn. None of this arcane medical knowledge was known when I graduated from medical school in 1975, so I have to hustle to keep up.

In fact, today as I walked with Oakley I relearned that little boys are made of "snips of snails and puppy dog tails". Oakley is different from my two daughters, who were of "sugar and spice and all things nice." I don't need a genetic analysis to see genetics at work as Oakley stomps through puddles and has to have a ball in his hand. And the learning goes on…

The Undiscovered Country - November 14, 2011

What do you say to someone who's just lost a loved one? You may be surprised to learn that it's not any easier for doctors, though they deal with tragedy every day. Mr. Jones routine office visit was not "routine" as he proceeded to tell me his forty-five year old wife had suddenly become sick and died. I've been treating him for depression, but he'd need more than my medication to see him through this *valley of the shadow of death,* let alone help him raise his two teenage boys.

I don't think anyone gets *over* the death of a loved one. About all we can do is navigate *around* the dark area placed in our life's journey. Many people fail to understand that the bereaving need our presence more than our philosophy. Platitudes often do more harm than good; showing up is much more important. Funerals are, after all, for the living rather than those who have *moved on to a new address.*

Two colleagues died last month. Both had lived long and rich lives before they began to weaken and finally relocated to what Shakespeare called the *undiscovered country.* My "granny" was your prototypical grandmother, and lived a hundred and two years. She was no philosopher, but as she weakened with age and disease, she once told me of her long life, "The first hundred were pretty good."

Of course we all want a life that is long and has quality, but if forced to choose most of us would opt for the latter over the former. The great fear is that we might linger in pain and debility, past a time when we're useful to ourselves and our families. The famous writer Earnest Hemingway was a self-described man's man. Yet, in his later years, Mr. Hemingway suffered through a long illness that he lamented "hurts so bad it takes away your dignity."

I've developed a prayer list for people I know, patients and the state of our country. This helps me focus beyond my own needs. Some believe that our reality is nothing but chance; I choose to think otherwise. A noted philosopher once observed that we humans will never understand God's ways, and I suspect he's right. I don't know why five of my patients are suffering from advanced cancer. I don't know why *Bad Things Happen to Good People*, the title of a book by Rabbi Kushner, where he writes of his son's progeria – accelerated and premature aging.

What I do know is that a faith perspective is helping the grieving Mr. Jones and several of my patients with cancer. I think prayer is like a group hug which makes the human creature feel less alone and more connected. The scholar and Christian apologist C. S. Lewis once said, "Prayer doesn't change the mind of God; it changes me." And many scientific papers have demonstrated that a faith perspective is associated with better outcomes that can't be explained by the healthier lifestyles of the faithful.

Recently, I was struck by the last words of Steve Jobs. At the end he was reported to have said, "Oh wow, oh wow." Thomas Edison perhaps also afforded us a glimpse in his last words, "It's beautiful over there." What did they see? Was their vision a dysfunction of their brains that doctors call delirium? Or was it narcotics that produced a false perception, a hallucination? We still know almost nothing about the *undiscovered country*.

A famous 17th century scientist named Blaise Pascal decided that his theories describing fluid mechanics (the basis of hydraulic brakes, etc.) were not as satisfying as the pursuit of God. He devoted the remainder of his life to spiritual issues. In his now famous *Pascal's Wager* he explains that it's a good bet to trust in God. Paraphrasing, Pascal said, if there is no God, when we die we blink into oblivion. However, if we trust in God, when we die we gain all – Socrates 2000 years earlier came to the same conclusion. I believe a faith perspective makes life better now, and there is the hope of then.

I'm a scientist and a realist. I deal in data such as blood counts and X-rays. I don't know everything and, in fact, a doctor who projects an all-knowing attitude is either already dangerous or soon will be. I now have a spiritual side that complements my logic and helps me serve my patients. I admit that I have little data to prove or disprove the existence of a greater reality, but I don't believe I deceive myself or mislead my patients when I apply the full extent of my science tempered by my faith.

After all it was Albert Einstein who said, "Religion without science is blind, but science without religion is lame." Well said, professor.

I just don't get it. I've been an observer of people and social mores for thirty-five years, and I just don't understand the whole vampire thing that seems to be sweeping the country. I was surprised when the books became the rage of the nurses at the hospital and the ladies in my office. And now the movie sequels with the young heart throbs Kristen Stewart and Robert Pattinson adorn the covers of magazines in the grocery check-out line.

My *consultants* assure me that the books are "so well written, Dr. Ferguson; and it's really a love story."

"But ladies," I say with tactful amazement, "the story involves vampires! How can you love a monster that's gnawing on your neck?"

I don't believe my argument had much sway with the *Twilight* devotees who just rolled their eyes wistfully as if to say that I just didn't understand. And I admit that I'm confused by this modern rendition of the Count Dracula legend. I've seen the old movies with Béla Lugosi and I loved Jack Nicholson in *Wolf*. Though I'm not a fan of horror flicks, I do think the old films had a certain degree of mystery associated with Transylvania and the Carpathian Mountains of Romania. And I have to admit that stories about vampires and werewolves are certainly better than the modern *Texas Chainsaw Massacre* horror films.

You might ask what any of this has to do with medicine. I think it has to do with the health of our society and the protection of our children. I'm for free speech, but some stories seem too intense for teeny boppers. Perhaps it's a cliché, but parents need to be wary of the effects of pop culture on their kids.

History has important lessons for us. In the tenth year of the Trojan War the besieged Trojans awakened one morning to find that the Greeks had left, and only a great horse remained that the Trojans thought was a tribute to their valorous defense of Troy. They rolled the giant inside the walls and well, you know the rest of the story.

I'm concerned about the influence that media and pop culture has on our people. I'm concerned that Sunday worship attendance is steadily declining. I'm worried that people see a spiritual perspective as irrelevant. I'm more fearful for my daughters and wife than I used to be, and I too am more careful given all the home invasions, robberies and rampant drug use in our dysfunctional culture. Now before you start to scream, I'm not equating the vampire craze with the mayhem in our streets. I'm opposed to censorship, but a shepherd watches out for his flock just as a watchman sounds the alarm if danger is perceived.

The general consensus is that these books and movies are truly love stories that have a happy ending, despite a love triangle between a vampire, a werewolf, and a human girl. The protagonist vampire is good because he and his kind only drink the blood of animals; it's the bad vampires who prey upon humans. Interestingly, the mission of the werewolves in this saga is to hunt down and destroy the bad vampires. Unfortunately, the girl is dying after a difficult child-vampire delivery, and has to be saved by a vampire transfusion. This transforms her into one of the "un-dead." Confused yet?

I have to admit that the actors in the movie are attractive people, and it is romantic that the actor Robert Pattison proposes on the movie set to Kristin Stewart. These actors seem more level headed than many in Hollywood and could be better role models than others from tinsel town.

I don't pretend to understand this phenomenon. After some research, I don't think the vampire craze is ghoulish or Goth or due to the attraction some young women seem to have for *bad boys*. I don't think it's about rebellion either; after all, humans are designed to push away from their parents and find their own way. But after reflection I remain uneasy and wonder if this craze is more than it seems superficially. I'm concerned about a Trojan horse.

Adults are capable of discriminating between right and wrong, but young people are still learning the lessons of life and we older folks are supposed to look out for them and impart values and wisdom. Sometimes young people listen; sometimes I didn't. But, something from my youth stuck with me, because during my *Dark Night of the Soul* (John of the Cross), I was able to fall back on the Way, and it made all the difference in my life.

The Proverbist said, "Point your kids in the right direction – when they're old they won't become lost." Wise words from long ago.

Travel is great, and it also makes you appreciate home. My medical partners coined the term "Ferg-isms" to describe my many aphorisms. One of these is "Get on a plane, rent a car and see the world." And Becky and I have been blessed to do so!

About once a year we go to my brother and sister-in-law's ranch in southwestern Colorado. There's a line from *Jeremiah Johnson,* an old western movie I like, where one of the characters refers to the Rocky Mountains as "the backbone of the world." You can imagine this looking up at the Milky Way high above the majestic San Juan Mountains that encircle Brother Bill's place.

The Rocky Mountains are geologic infants compared to our Appalachian Mountains. About 450 million years ago our Smoky Mountains were formed from the collision of tectonic plates and once may have been even more majestic than the 14,000 foot Rockies. However, water and wind are powerful forces and they eroded our mountains, making them rounded and very different from the lofty Rocky Mountain spikes.

The beauty of the high mountain country swept over me as Becky, my brother Steve and I hiked to the top of a waterfall above the town of Telluride, Colorado. It was a perfect day with the deep blue skies seen at elevations of 11,000 feet. The quaking aspens, rushing streams, and the towering mountains made me think deeply and vastly. I sensed John Denver's *Rocky Mountain High.*

We descended from our mountaintop *high* to mosey the streets of Telluride and watch our ladies shop. Thankfully, sidewalk benches are provided for men folk. There are new stores in Telluride this year. With the legalization of "medicinal marijuana" a new industry has sprung up with multiple new clinics offering their services. In fact, there are now more *marijuana clinics* than liquor stores and coffee shops in Telluride.

One member of my family was approached by a young lady and, after some chit-chat, the twenty-something said she was "recruiting" for the clinic. She offered to escort my sister-in-law to the clinic and help her log on to the video-doctor who would undoubtedly approve her for a medicinal marijuana prescription. Sis declined, telling the young sales-person that her lumbago wasn't that bad.

That evening as my family gathered to cook supper and enjoy a glass of wine we discussed the Rocky Mountain *high* this clinic was hawking. Even the *Telluride Magazine* had advertisements for the clinics. An article in Telluride's newspaper quoted a local who opined that the "*Cana-business* is going to bring our economy back, [since] in a ski town like this there's a lot of joint pain."

Those of us in Tennessee find it strange that fellow Americans in Colorado and seven other states allow the medicinal use of cannabis that violates federal laws. What a contrast to our neighboring Hawkins County where the sheriff recently found and uprooted 500 marijuana plants yesterday in Rogersville.

There is some science behind the use of medicinal marijuana in cancer patients undergoing chemotherapy, especially if there is intractable nausea and vomiting. Also, there is some data to suggest the use of cannabis in certain AIDS syndromes and glaucoma patients. What concerns me is the obvious abuse advertised and hawked in Telluride. I'm concerned about the risk of psychoactive chemicals as an entry drug to ever more problematic agents; and my psychiatric consultants agree with my concerns. I also realize that it is virtually impossible to outlaw the use of a naturally occurring substance. After all, we Americans repealed *prohibition*.

Perhaps I'm libertarian in my philosophy regarding these *natural* agents; just don't ask me or others to clean up the mess you make of your life by abusing drugs. And despite statements by aficionados that marijuana has been used since the third century BC and is legal in nine other countries, I find the thought of inhaling any smoke distasteful and potentially carcinogenic. And who is regulating the cannabis content of brownies?

In final analysis I have concerns that we need chemicals to live well. And I believe we must protect our children until they are mature enough to make wise decisions for themselves, and be able to accept the consequences of their choices. I can't see the medicinal value of cannabis cooking oil, cookies, snack crackers or canna-butter. And I may never eat out again in Telluride after seeing the chef exit the clinic.

I guess you'd say I prefer a natural Rocky Mountain High!

Somehow in the midst of all the turmoil, life goes on and renews itself. On May Day my grandson arrived, and things seem brighter now. Yes, the destruction continues in Washington, wars rage around the world and injustice is even encountered in our city government. But, now a new star shines among us and hope returns.

My mother's father was a carpenter and sometimes went by the name, T.O., short for Thomas Oakley Burleson. I have a picture of him holding me high above his head in the first months of my life. And clearly visible is the twinkle in his eye and a broad smile of delight across his face. I don't have a comparative picture of me holding my grandson above my head, at least not yet; he's a neonate and is too young for calisthenics, and it might make my daughter faint.

We're especially protective of our firstborn. My grandson does share something with Jenny's great-grandfather, and for that matter my son-in-law's grandfather as well. You see, my grandson is their namesake, Oakley Augustine Johnson. And when Oakley squeezes my finger I'm convinced he'll be as strong as oaken wood and as brilliant as St. Augustine.

We all have "gifts differing" observed the Apostle Paul. This champion of the Christian message was a learned man, a theologian, and a philosopher. I suspect he was also a keen observer of the differences between the sexes. Have you ever wondered why men can't find things? Or, have you ever considered why women are physically and emotionally softer? However, it's a misconception to think that compassion and empathy are signs of weakness.

Women are the glue of society. You can quote me on that. I have some talents, but my nurturing skills pale in comparison to women in general and my wife's in particular. Men would be savages without the tempering influences of the women around us. And now I see my daughter in a new light growing in grace as she holds and nurtures Oakley, and balances the men in her family.

I remember some years ago a somewhat frantic call from my mother. She said that my father was limping and the back brace his chiropractor neighbor had sold him wasn't helping his misery. I drove my father to my office and after examining him I told him that his problem wasn't sciatica. Though my parents put me through medical school, my father was no fan of the medical profession. Perhaps because he was in such misery, he finally agreed to a cortisone injection into his inflamed knee. His pain miraculously abated and on the way home he told me how he now saw me in a new light. It didn't matter that I was married with two kids and had a thriving medical practice. The point is it's hard for parents to see their kids as anything but their children. But fortunately, my girls still see me as their daddy; and that's a blessing.

I find that I am less fearful of the future these days. Most of my milestones have been reached. I do worry about our country and the parallels I see in the lessons of history. I worry that The Spirit is seen as irrelevant to so many and that the inevitable void is being filled by idols and the State. Mostly, I have concerns about my girls, and now my grandson.

Times were tough during the Depression years when my grandparents were trying to hold things together gardening and selling eggs door-to-door in more affluent Sequoyah Hills. My life has been, by comparison, a breeze. I've told Becky many times that if I died today, "It's been a good run." Now, don't get me wrong, I've got lots of life left in me, taking care of my patients, developing our property, writing, and now I have a new reason to carry on – Oakley.

Everyone thinks their child is the cutest and special; and of course they're right. This week's "Piaget" teaching point is the next time someone wants to show you pictures of their child or grandchild, be glad that there's a parent and family who loves that kid enough to carry pictures and brag a bit. Too many kids don't have someone to love them or to *hold'em high*.

If you want to save the world start with your family, and follow the advice of the Proverbist in chapter 22:6: "Teach children how they should live and they will remember it all their life." My teacher's role has just been extended to another generation.

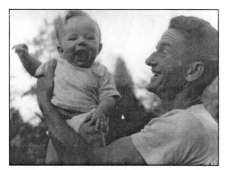

JD held high by Oakley Burleson
(1951)

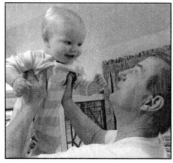

Oakley Johnson held high by JD
(2012)

Ethnicity has little to do with rhythm because my grandson Noah has it. We don't know where he got it because my son-in-law doesn't dance. Perhaps it's some recessive or ancestral gene that courses through Noah's blood and allows him to move like no white man I've ever seen.

Sitting on the beach watching and hearing the ocean's waves makes me think about the rhythms of life. Our bodies operate with a daily (diurnal) rhythm defined by the sun. Light rays stimulate not only our retinas, but also the pineal gland which produces melatonin that influences our sleep cycle. When we travel across multiple time zones our bodies have trouble adjusting, producing "jet-lag" because our pineal gland's melatonin production is out of synch.

"Where do waves come from?" I asked Mr. Google, as I sat watching and listening to the crashing Atlantic surf. Lots of things interest me, and the same inquisitive perspective led the ancient Greeks to a scientific study of the world around them. They called this desire to know things "gnosis", the root word for our word knowledge. I believe if you ever lose your inquisitiveness you will rapidly become obsolete. I tell patients to beware of the doctor who implies that he's always right, because it often means he's closed his mind to further learning and will soon be dangerous, if he isn't already.

Waves are largely created by the wind. When the sun heats the air it rises, and cooler air blows in to fill the relative void. As the air moves across the water it causes a dragging force along the surface pulling the water upward. The result is a rolling tsunami-like swell. Stronger winds over greater distances produce bigger waves which ultimately encounter the beach. The water at the bottom of a wave is slowed by the rising shore causing the wave to topple over in a crash of surf.

We live in a world of sound which we take for granted until it dissipates or is lost. Many of my patients become increasingly isolated as they lose their hearing and can mistakenly appear dull. The sound of surf occurs when ocean wave energy is changed into sound waves that move through the air and are channeled into the ear canal. At the end of the canal is the ear drum which is moved backwards and forwards by sound waves. This movement, in turn, causes the three conductive bones of the middle ear to function like a piston and pump another drum-like apparatus on the cochlea. It is the resulting movement of fluid waves in this hearing organ that stimulates nerve signals which race to the brain where they are interpreted as crashing surf.

A Philosopher named George Berkeley once said that a tree falling in the forest makes no sound if no one is there to hear the falling tree. What he meant was that sound is interpretive. There may be sound energy produced when a tree crashes to the forest floor, but if no one is there to hear the crash, there's no sound. Hmm, I'll leave that to your reflection and return to practicality.

Sounds come intermittently and rhythmically. They also come at different energies and frequencies. A man's voice is deeper because testosterone elongates his larynx producing his Adam's apple. The longer vocal chords produce a deeper voice. No one can deny that teenage girls produce a piecing high frequency sound.

Sounds also come to us as intensity or loudness. I read that crashing waves can produce sound energy measured at 70 decibels (dB) and is comparable to automobile traffic. A faint sound like rustling leaves registers 20 dBs whereas a quiet library is 30-40 dBs. Human conversation occurs in the 50-60 dB range. The Seinfeld sitcom once spoofed people who talk so softly as to be misheard. That's not the same as the inarticulate mumble of your teenage son or when my wife says I didn't listen; the latter is due to the Y chromosome! Lawn mowers produce damaging 90 dB sound energy. I learned that sporting events like a Tennessee Volunteer football game generates 110 dB cheers comparable to rock concerts and jet planes. Guns and jack hammers produce 130-140 dB concussions and obviously require hearing protection. Ear plugs and ear muffs do help, but decrease sound energy about 30 dBs.

There's something primordial about relentless waves on a beach. They make me think of other rhythms of life. I don't often think about breathing. The non-conscious area of my brain is tasked to control respiration, heartbeat, blood pressure and even digestive processes. In fact, these processes work best when the conscious brain leaves them alone. I often see patients who sense "breathlessness" when their anxiety spills over into their subconscious systems.

Most of us have lain awake at night and been unable to sleep. Who hasn't worried about something and tried to "force" sleep on a system designed to induce sleep, if we'd just leave it alone? Sometimes I find it helpful to listen to my rhythmic breathing in the middle of the night. Like ocean waves, this primordial rhythm of life seems to be a better distraction than counting sheep.

It's time to exit my beach musings, but I'll leave you with two additional rhythms to consider. The first comes from my Master through Eugene Peterson's translation, The Message. Jesus said, "Come away with me and you'll recover your life... Learn the unforced rhythms of Grace" (Matthew 11:28-30). The second comes from The Prophet by Khalil Gibran who wrote, "And what is it to cease breathing, but to free the breath from its restless tides, that it may rise and expand and seek God unencumbered?"
Food for thought...

I'll probably get in trouble with my Mother because of this title. She hates it when I suggest I'm getting old. Perhaps I should have named the story **Older** Dogs and New Tricks. I actually like where I am in my life, but I might as well because I can't change time's effects on my body, only my attitude. I've asked lots of people if they'd like to be sixteen years old again. We'd all like to have more youthful bodies where everything works, but invariably people say "No" to going back and having to learn the hard lessons of life over again.

Last Saturday I learned a new trick as I accompanied my daughter, son-in-law, and wife to my first farm equipment auction. Who would have thought that I would be in the market for a bush hogging machine to drag behind the Massey-Ferguson tractor we'd bought the week before? Obviously I was out of my element strolling down the rows of strange looking machines with various shades of red, green, mustard and rust. Fortunately, my son-in-law knew what he was doing and educated me on the finer aspects of used farm equipment. And when the bidding was done I found myself with a bush-hogger that we named *Rusty,* for obvious reasons. I'm already picturing myself as Oliver Douglas from **Green Acres** astride my tractor.

My daughter and son-in-law are working with us to develop our property into a place for themselves and their horses. Becky and I think this is a grand idea, but it will take lots of work and some serious machinery to clear the trees and brush.

You might ask what this has to do with a medical column. Well, this whole process has caused me to reconsider nuclear and extended family concepts. We hear a lot these days about the tough economy and twenty-somethings moving back home with parents. They even made a movie about the *failure to launch* condition where kids don't grow up and accept the mantle of adult responsibility.

I once read a marvelous book called **Cold Sassy Tree**. The story begins with the matriarch of the family dying from complications of a stroke. The story takes place in Georgia, circa 1905, in a world vastly different from our own. There wasn't much you could do for a stroke then and people were cared for at home among loved ones instead of in high tech hospitals. Many believe that hospital environments isolate us from the realities of our mortality. However, for me the book was most noteworthy for the multigenerational living arrangements of the early 1900s. Years ago kids grew up with grandparents in the home and amidst their accumulated wisdom of life's lessons. Eastern cultures revere their older citizens with the *venerable* moniker. Japan's Shintoism even worships its deceased and honored ancestors.

I don't mean to go nostalgic on you because there were tough times in early America as there are now. I wouldn't want to go back to a time when there weren't antibiotics, indoor plumbing and baths only on Saturday night. It does concern me that in a few generations we've gone from a people who were pretty self-sufficient to a civilization so complex and specialized that I don't believe we could provide for ourselves if there was a sustained disruption of our modern supply lines.

What I'm really looking forward to is my daughter's family moving next door to us, though not in with us. Becky and I are lucky that both our girls are *launched* and doing well. But it's great that we're still a part of their lives, and even better when we can help them with a project that will bring us closer together. Who knows, maybe I'll like becoming a gentleman farmer on our *green-acres* among grandchildren.

And I'm looking forward to learning how to operate Leroy, my son-in-law's name for our tractor. In the meantime, I'll just provide you with a picture of me sitting atop our tractor. There's more to me than internal medicine and geriatrics!

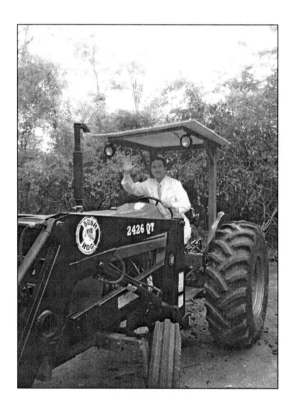

The Misery of a Cold - February 9, 2010

I kept telling myself that I wasn't going to die, but as I drove to the Emergency Room last Saturday night to see an even sicker patient, I wasn't sure that I was going to make it. A patient once told me the *flu* made him so sick he was afraid he wouldn't die. I understand hyperbole and perhaps I'm being a bit dramatic, but it's been a tough week, a really long weekend on-call, and I really feel awful.

"Doctors aren't supposed to get sick," patients kept telling me as I made hospital rounds and did my best to care for those worse off than me. I was touched by these folks with truly life-threatening illnesses, who were still able to empathize with their Doc who was suffering along with them. Even the ER Staff – who normally steels themselves emotionally to the endless stream of suffering around them – was sympathetic.

"You look terrible, Dr. Ferguson, and sound even worse," said my friend, nurse Nan. "Have you seen a doctor?"

I mumbled agreement with her assessment, as I scanned the lab data of the patient I had been called to evaluate.

"Nan, if I had a cure for this cold I'd be rich and famous and I wouldn't be in the ER especially during the Alabama/Tennessee football game."

I often tell young doctors that if they live long enough they'll have many of the afflictions of their patients, and this will teach them empathy. Unfortunately, they often look at me in a vacuous way, tilting their heads quizzically like my dog does as he tries to triangulate a strange sound in the yard. The ancient Greeks had a philosophy that wisdom only comes about through suffering.

Their point was that experience is the great teacher. I've never had cancer or a heart attack or any number of other life threatening problems, but I am well acquainted with the feverish misery of a bad cold and having to suck it up and get the job done. Parents especially know what I mean, and so did my patients who appreciated my efforts, especially because of my obvious misery.

Experts say there are more than eighty cold producing viruses. I don't know which one I had, but it was a nasty one. As I made rounds I was especially careful to wash my hands and use hand sanitizers, while holding my breath as I examined patients. As you know, colds are spread by sneezed or coughed droplets, or by contact with contaminated hands. I repeatedly told staff members to go wash their hands after they laid sympathetic hands on my shoulders. I told them "I wouldn't give this misery to my worst enemy, let alone you."

I even started to worry about my dog, Jack, who is always trying to kiss me with his tongue. I asked an infectious disease colleague whether dogs get colds; and he didn't know. Maybe when I'm better I'll research the subject with some of my patients who are veterinarians at the University of Tennessee Vet Center.

So how do you manage a cold? Here are some common sense guidelines. You should see your doctor immediately if you have a bad cold with a high fever, since this may be Influenza. You should see your doctor if a cold lasts longer than seven days or begins to improve only to again worsen with new symptoms and suggests a complication.

Unfortunately, there's not a lot modern science can do for the majority of cold syndromes except provide comfort treatment. Rest is advisable, but sometimes is not an option. Decongestants can help head congestion. Expectorants help to keep bronchial mucous from becoming thick and ropey. And never underestimate the value of chicken soup, a hot toddy or a sympathetic touch.

This is a time of Thanksgiving, and I am thankful for so many things. Becky and I love all aspects of the Holiday Season, from Thanksgiving through Christmas.

I'm especially thankful for my patients who give me purpose and so many stories! My wife's cousin admits that he gets all his stories from the news and his readers – kind of like the stories my patients give me.

I have the utmost respect for my patients, but as Art Linkletter once said about kids, they can "say the darndest things."

Our office had to purchase headsets for our nurses taking telephone messages, primarily because people walking past the nurse's station were overhearing patient's concerns that I can't begin to relate to you; some would be X-rated.

Perhaps it's good that patients trust us and confide in us. We all just have to be careful in these days of the internet and Facebook. Recently, one of my patients suffered a heart attack, and a cardiac arrest. Fortunately, he was resuscitated and was saved by cardiac stenting of a blocked artery. I learned about his crisis when the details were posted by his son on the social networking Facebook system! And his son is a doctor! Generation X's and Millenials certainly look at the world differently than the Boomers or the Greatest Generation.

My patient, Mrs. Jones, was seeing me for a physical exam, and after pleasantries I left the room so that she could disrobe and put on a paper gown. My nurse and I explain to women that the paper top is to be open in the back rather than the front, but nine times out of ten arrange the opening in the front. I asked myself for years why patients did this, and then it hit me. Gynecologists always ask ladies to arrange their gowns open in the front, and since gynecologic exams are... sensitive, patients have been conditioned as teenagers and young women to don their gowns in a certain way; it's hard to overcome imprinted routines.

I was doing phone messages with my nurse as I waited for Mrs. Jones, when I heard a scream. Rushing to her exam room I saw the poor lady clutching her inadequate paper garments around her as she attempted to cover up. None of us had anticipated she would be *flashing* anyone four stories up.

You might be thinking of a peeping Tom with a telescope or binoculars. You'd be wrong. Never underestimate a window washer's ability to scale tall buildings.

Doctors can get embarrassed even though clinical exams are not sexual. Ms. Smith was a croupier by profession. She was an attractive lady, but considered her bust to be insufficient to garner the tips she might otherwise command if she possessed better cleavage. She asked my opinion and I told her that she was healthy and if the augmentation would make her feel better about herself, then she should proceed. I saw her again sometime later for a physical and she was quite pleased with her surgery... no, she was proud of her new look. I instructed her on the paper gown routine and left the room allowing her to get ready for the exam.

I always knock before entering a patient's exam or hospital room. As I knocked, Ms. Smith said she was ready. As I entered the room there she stood in all her glory in a contrapposto stance with arms outstretched in a runway wave. She said, "What'd ya think, Doc?" Can you picture a man in a white coat attempting the back stroke to maneuver toward the safety of the hallway?

Our office is going through a lot of changes lately and it has started me thinking about the endgame strategy. I'm not ready to retire because I now picture myself in the Indian summer of my life and career. I enjoy my life and believe in what I do. So, for the time being I'm concentrating on the Brother Lawrence perspective. I still have lots to give before I lay it all down. And were I to quit, where would I get my stories??

It was dawn and I was wide awake because we had gone to bed so early. No wonder Ben Franklin's invention of bifocals was so important; it's tough to read by candlelight. I'm just glad the storms and the power outages were only an inconvenience and a temporary respite from the internet and cable news. Candlelight is kind of cozy for awhile; I can't say the same for cold showers.

The storms that blew through the South were unparalleled since the 1974 super-cell that spawned over two hundred tornados. At last count the recent storms that destroyed Tuscaloosa and killed more than 300 people across the South generated over 300 tornadoes, including an F1 that struck our south Knoxville area. I didn't see the tornado that turned great trees in our neighborhood into toothpicks, but we did experience *bodacious* hailstones the size of plums. I love the word bodacious, made famous by our friend David Keith in the movie **An Officer and a Gentleman**.

In the growing light I went out to survey the damage that was thankfully minimal. What struck me most was the cheerful chirping and singing of birds in the aftermath of hail that turned the hoods of cars into beaten metal, knocked out windows, and shredded my garden and roses. How could there be any birds alive after that bombardment, I asked myself and others? I know that if I had been out in the forest without protection I would have been beaten to death.

We have such an anthropomorphic (the word for the week) vision of the Universe. We think what happens to mankind is of utmost cosmological significance. And maybe it is. Perhaps our beautiful planet is an aberration and there are no other places of similar wonder which promote and sustain thoughtful life. However, in February 2011, NASA reported that its *Kepler Planet Hunter* has now identified over 1,200 planets, some approximately the size of our Earth.

For some time we've known of the ever-increasing number of huge planets circling distant stars, but it's hard to imagine earthlike environments in planets the size of our own Jupiter. Some of these newer smaller planetoids are even in the so-called habitable zone where life like ours could conceivably occur.

Are we alone in the Universe? My first novel, *Epiphany*, a science fiction yarn, asked this fundamental question. My answer was no. I don't think the Creator would make thoughtful life on only one planet, circling one average star, in the outer rim of one average galaxy, among the 100 billion other known galaxies of the Universe. I don't mean to be heretical, but what a waste of space if we're alone.

Since the Universe is so big I don't believe there will be travel to another star and or any of these newly discovered planets in my lifetime. So, I'll remain content on this beautiful planet that we call Earth and home. Yes, nature can be savage and tragedy unpredictable, but there is also wonder and majesty. And a part of this wonder is the human creature which the Psalmist described as "fearfully and wonderfully made." However, with less lofty verbiage I sometimes quip to my patients that I didn't design their marvelous aching bodies; I just work on 'em.

There's much I don't understand about tornados, hurricanes and the hearts of men. And I don't know why bad things sometimes happen to seemingly good people. I've just learned to trust that the morning light will bring back birdsong after the storm.

"The world stands out on either side, no wider than the heart is wide;
Above the world is stretched the sky, no higher than the soul is high..."

Edna St. Vincent Millay

I think it's easier to comprehend the vastness of the ocean (and the world) from the deck of a ship. Our seagoing home is huge and is shared with three thousand other souls, yet it bobs like a cork on an ocean that stretches to the horizon and for three and a half miles beneath us.

Becky and I are not "boat people," but I needed to get away and she knew I needed R&R, rescue from the world and restoration of the soul. Thankfully, there are last minute cruise deals, so here I sit contemplating clouds so low you can almost touch them and a kaleidoscopic of Caribbean colors.

You can't ignore colors in the Caribbean. Perhaps it's the sun and light that causes people to choose bright and vibrant colors over somber choices of higher latitudes. Darkness is, after all, the absence of light. The 19th century French Impressionist painters understood the importance of light, though I doubt Monet considered the physics of electromagnetic radiation from our sun.

Our ability to see color is dependent on light energy of a certain spectrum which activates photoreceptors in the retina of our eyes. When I was a boy I was taught the mnemonic ROY G BIV which describes the colors we see as revealed by a prism. Red, orange, and yellow colors are associated with the longer, less energetic, wave lengths of light energy. Blue, indigo, and violet colors are found in the shorter wavelengths of electromagnetic radiation. Verdant colors are found as we shift from the red to the blue end of the visible spectrum.

The physics of light brings such beauty and wonder to those who have eyes to see. Some people don't stop to consider yellow daffodils, and others are color blind and see differently. My father-in-law had red-green color blindness. He was once asked what red looks like to him. He replied to his interlocutor, "Well, what does it look like to you?" The point is you can't describe "red;" it must be experienced.

There are practical aspects of physics beyond just science and esthetics. Most of us have observed the rising tone of an ambulance as it approaches. This occurs because the sound waves are compressed as the ambulance approaches resulting in a rising frequency of sound and an increasing tenor. Similarly, as the ambulance recedes, the tone of the siren decreases as the sound wave is stretched and the frequency of sound energy decreases. This is called the Doppler Effect, and it applies to light waves as well as sound energy.

The 20th century astronomer, Edmund Hubble, noted that the color spectrum in sequential photographs of stars was shifted toward the red end of the spectrum, and he concluded that virtually all stars in the Universe are moving away from us. This was a paradigm shift from our notion that the Universe was vast, but fixed. Hubble's observation has been repeatedly confirmed and is offered as proof that our Universe continues to expand from its origin 13.5 billion years ago.

Becky has tried to explain the color wheel to me before, but it finally "sunk in" from the deck of our ship. The color wheel came up in our conversation because I was intrigued why orange seaweed floating upon a deep blue sea was so appealing to my senses.

Diagram:

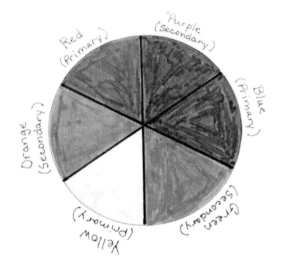

And that's when my lesson began.

Becky explained that when a red, blue or yellow primary color is matched with a secondary color on the opposite side of the color wheel "it works and is visually pleasing."

"You're right!" I exclaimed. (I always try to agree with my wife.)

We see the world through the three primary colors and their blends as depicted on the color wheel diagram. We find it esthetically pleasing when an object reflects the wavelengths of a primary color juxtaposed to its complementary color. Orange works with blue, and the red and green of Christmas is likewise pleasing. Fellows, esthetics has its place and a Big Orange tie with a red shirt is garish. In fact, another group of French painters were known as the *Fauves* because they used garish colors and were described as painting like "*wild dogs*."

The eye is a wondrous organ and has been called the window of the soul by poets. A picture of the sea or a story can never capture the beauty or grandeur of the world. Sometimes we need to slow down and consider the beauty around us as did William Wordsworth as he gazed and then reflected on a field of yellow daffodils:

*"...I gazed and gazed but little thought what joy to me that crowd had brought: For oft, when on my couch I lie in vacant or in pensive mood, they flash upon that **inward eye** which is the bliss of solitude. And then my heart with pleasure fills, and dances with the daffodils."*

Veterans Day - November 17, 2008

We gathered in the Veterans' Cemetery Octagon to honor a hero whose time had come. I knew he was a hero because I had been his doctor for more than twenty years. Over time you come to know the patients you serve, but I'm frequently surprised when I see them in different contexts. (We've all been flummoxed running into an acquaintance in a different setting.)

We doctors try to educate our patients, diagnose their problems and control their medical conditions, but with Bert the best I could do was damage control. Fortunately, he was a tough guy and *finished the race,* leading his family and teaching me a thing or two about life along the way.

As I sat there in the Veterans' Cemetery listening to his son and others remember this "big strong marine," my thoughts drifted back to a cold but bright February morning in 1996. We gathered in the same place for a similar military funeral service, that time held in honor of my Dad who was a navy hero. In fact, as I think about how fate or purpose plays out, it is somewhat of a miracle that I am here to pen these words. You see my Dad was a naval aviator on the aircraft carrier *Yorktown* three days out of Pearl Harbor on December 7, 1941. The Japanese were looking for a carrier that Sunday morning, but had to settle for the *Arizona* and other battleships. Had the attack been a few days later, I probably wouldn't be here to reflect on Veterans' Day, Bert or my dad, whose tombstone now lies among thousands of other veterans who so nobly gave of themselves in the cause of freedom and the ideals of the United States of America.

This was my second funeral of the week. It seems that they come more often now as my cohort of contemporaries age. I've always heard it said that funerals are for the living. We gather to support the grieving family and to celebrate a life well-lived. Most importantly, funerals are a time for reflection on relationships – all the connections, and the things shared and remembered. We participants learn a lot from those who leave us. What a privilege to see people in a light that sometimes only comes with shared remembrances.

After Bert's service had ended, I searched for my Father's gravesite, scanning the tombstones spread over the hillside above Northshore Drive, I thought about all those people who lived and loved and who are now gone, though remembered here in this place of honor. What were their stories and family traditions?

I've often regretted that I never served in the military. Most veterans speak so highly of the lessons of honor, duty and country, learned as a result of their military years. My Dad spoke of how transformative that period was for him. Bert's son said the same as he eulogized his Father. As I watched the honor guards salute Bert with a twenty-one gun salute, I again found myself envious of the camaraderie and respect engendered through sacrifice for country and creed.

We all will die; it is inevitable. I've observed that young people sometimes take such chances with their lives, perhaps because for them death is far away in the future and merely a vague concept. We older people know differently; maybe that's why it's the young who go off to war. To those of us old enough to have seen parents get sick and die or see friends keel over, death is real to us. I now understand why my Mother always told me to be careful as I headed out the door seeking adventure.

Elizabeth Kubler Ross wrote the sentinel work on dying and death in the 1960s. Dr. Ross noted five stages: disbelief, bargaining, anger, depression, and acceptance. I didn't have to go through those stages for Bert or for my Father; these men lived long and large. Like Greek heroes they live on in the minds of all of those who knew them.

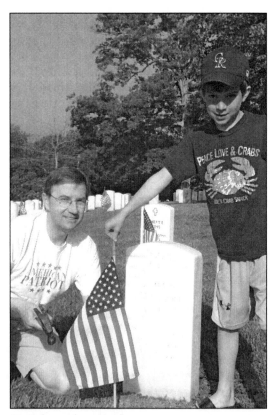

JD and grandson Noah

54

The Meaning of Life - June 24, 2011

A man by the name of Viktor Frankl once said "Striving to find meaning in one's life is the primary motivational force in man." You may not have heard of Dr. Frankl, but he survived Auschwitz and other Nazi death camps during WW II, and went on to found the Third Viennese School of Psychotherapy called Logotherapy.

Dr. Frankl has what I call *street creds*. He has "walked the walk," and has earned the right to tell his story and offer his conclusions. I'm certainly not an expert in the Freudian, Adlerian or any other school of psychotherapy – though I dabble in what makes people work and why they founder. A good clinician has to treat the whole person and not just the body.

Sometimes diseases occur when we fail to do the things which promote health such as eating correctly and avoiding tobacco. However, I'm increasingly aware that genetics affect all human functions and sometimes diseases occur because of the genetic tendencies we inherit. In recent years scientists have been able to map the entire human genome – the blue print human life. There was great fanfare that this monumental scientific discovery would soon translate into affordable gene analysis which could predict disease. Unfortunately, it's much more complicated than this simplistic description and hope.

There are some well-known examples where a certain genetic type will inevitably cause a disease. The singer Arlo Guthrie finally decided to see if he carried the gene that produced Huntington's Dementia in his father Woody Guthrie. Arlo did not inherit his father's gene and will be spared his father's neurodegenerative disease. But this generating technology raises ethical concerns. Would you want to know that your destiny is dementia at fifty years old, given that there is no cure? Would this knowledge make you live your life differently?

Actually there's a simpler, more pragmatic and less expensive way to predict disease. It's called taking a careful family history of the patient's relatives. If everyone in your family develops coronary artery disease in their fifties, you should be aware of your increased risk, but remember risk is not inevitability. And if everyone in your family lives into their nineties, you might be less concerned by a cholesterol reading of two hundred and fifty mg/dl.

Dr. Frankl admits that he was fortunate to survive the Holocaust and its death camps. In reading his story I glean that his character and his sense of purpose afforded him hope and the desire to live. The Apostle Paul wrote similarly of perseverance, character and hope in his epistle to the Romans two thousand years ago.

Recently, I was challenged by my minister's sermon when he observed that, "Life has no meaning in itself." His message was a reference to the human need for relationship with God, but I believe there is similarity with the writings of Paul and Dr. Frankl, and what I see as a growing sense of purposelessness in our country.

I'm troubled to encounter more and more people who seemingly have no faith in God, or so little that they have become "functional" atheists. Instead, they place their hope in the institutions of man. Our evolving welfare system is an example. Though once well intentioned, it now crushes personal responsibility and replaces the integral and timeless notion of Deity with State. In a sense we have created a modern equivalent of the *Golden Calf* idol. And it's not just the Government that people expect to care for them. The same philosophy is operative in our hospitals where people show up in the ER without a personal physician to be their advocate or direct their hospital care. Disturbingly, people trust the system or whoever is on call to look out for them in their hour of greatest need.

I'm concerned about the abrogation of personal responsibility in so many aspects of our culture. The freedom to choose must be associated with good *and* bad consequences, just like the lessons we are supposed to be teaching our children. I have to admit that I'm more than frustrated when people make bad choices and then expect forgiveness with a public apology and a tearful appearance on Oprah's show. I once heard a story regarding expectations. It goes, "To an Irishman death is imminent. To an Englishman death is inevitable. But to an American death is negotiable." Folks, modern science and technology have limits. We can't reverse a lifetime of poor choices, and we don't have the ability or the wisdom to alter a person's DNA.

There is no such thing as *fairness* in the Universe. Fairness, like justice is a human notion, though a noble one. The best we can hope for is equal opportunity under law; equality is an idyllic illusion of man.

So what is the meaning or purpose in life? The writer of Ecclesiastes discovered the purpose of life. I recommend you consider this wisdom writing. In the meantime I'll share with you my simpler version. Meaning it is found in the three Fs: faith, family, and friends, and through a lifetime of service to others and country.

Travel Trilogy:
*Most of my essays are intended to stand alone though recurring themes are inevitable. However, the next three essays are companion pieces and therefore placed together as a "travelogue." My weekly newspaper column is entitled **The Doctor Is In**. I began this series with the title, **The Doctor Is Not In**!*

Bucket Trip - September 9, 2013

By the time you read this essay I'll be long gone. No, I've not eloped, the medical term for patients who choose a stairwell exit to escape from their hospital confines. Nor have I run off to a monastery fleeing the problems of our country. And I've not contracted some terminal illness. Mark Twain once quipped, "The news of my death has been greatly exaggerated." I'm not dead, just 5500 miles away on a Homeric adventure like Odysseus.

I wanted to stand on Athens' Acropolis one more time and reflect upon the ancient Athenian Greeks who gave the world its first democracy. Our word democracy comes from the Greek word demokratia, constructed from demos (the people) and kratia which in English becomes -cracy and means rule or power.

The Athenian democracy was far from perfect. The imperfect ancient Greeks even practiced infanticide and slavery was commonplace and the accepted norm. The Athenian democracy excluded women because citizenship was dependent on military service which was only an option for men in that patriarchal era. Perhaps military service should again be a prerequisite for politicians who are responsible for sending our sons and daughters in harm's way.

I wanted to sail the Adriatic like Virgil's legendary Aeneas who escaped Troy's destruction and migrated to Italy with his comrades. Together, with the Latin people, Rome was founded. I wanted to sail along the Dalmatian coast of the former Yugoslavia and see Dubrovnik, Croatia, the "Pearl of the Adriatic." I wanted to spend our thirty-eighth wedding anniversary in Venice at the "top" of the Adriatic, and sit in Saint Mark's Square a last time. And for twenty-five years I've dreamed of seeing the Sistine Chapel in Rome finally cleaned of the soot and grime of centuries to reveal the color-filled palate of the great Renaissance master Michelangelo.

You now have my itinerary and my plan is something of a travelogue. Some complain when I'm not discussing some arcane medical topic in my column. My reply is there's plenty of time and columns for vertigo, arthritis and such. Bucket trips are sentinel events and I write about my *focus* of the moment. The Kramer character on Seinfeld was once asked about his upcoming trip to California. He told Jerry Seinfeld that he was apparently like me "already there" (in his mind). As we packed, I thought about a column I once wrote entitled "Emporiatrics." This branch of internal medicine deals with the health issues of travel. You wouldn't need a travel specialist for a trip to Ooltewah, Tennessee, but foreign travel is another matter. So are the physiologic issues of prolonged airplane flights. Most people know that a cramped seat in coach increases the risks of blood clots, and a travel expert would recommend getting up and walking around every few hours during a long flight. When I get up to use the restroom I also do some deep knee bends waiting for the loo or in the galley to get my blood pumping in my legs.

Did you know that airplane cabins are only pressurized to the equivalent of 8000 feet above sea level? The reduced oxygen level can pose a significant risk to people with lung or heart disease. However, high altitude problems can occur in healthy people who travel to Machu Picchu, or who visit Leadville, Colorado in our Rocky Mountains.

Some years ago Becky and I rafted the Colorado River through the Grand Canyon. I learned then that the tamarisk tree is an Old World shrub that invaded the Canyon and is replacing the natural flora. Planes and ships have allowed foreign species to migrate to areas that would otherwise be inaccessible. It works for people as well who think nothing of taking a safari on the Serengeti Plains of Africa. Though our ancestors lived there long ago, we people of North America are now at risk for diseases of the Old World if we travel there without vaccinations and prophylactic medications. I advise people to see me with their travel itinerary rather than consulting the Health Department nurse. Sometimes patients take my advice.

Travel to Western Europe doesn't pose unusual risks for Americans aside from colds transmitted by fellow travelers through the re-circulated air system of airplanes. Our group of travelers will undoubtedly experience some "jet lag" as we travel across many time zones, and I never sleep well in a cramped seat with folks walking around all the time. A friend of a friend's recipe for the Atlantic crossing consists of 10 milligrams of Valium, followed by a *sleeping pill* and chased with four alcoholic highballs. Actually, I consider his "travel cocktail" ill advised, and I think this guy has a serious drug problem. Another trans-Atlantic traveler confided in me that she took an Ambien after two glasses of wine and passed out (or went to sleep) waiting in line for the restroom to empty. She's lucky she didn't break her hip and end up in a Paris hospital like another patient of mine who wrecked her Segway seeing the City of Lights. The only lights she saw were stars as she crashed to the pavement.

I believe travel broadens one's perspective, and if you have the itch to travel, you should. After all, you can play it safe and then fall out of your rocker on the front porch and break your hip. I only have one reservation regarding my Bucket Trip. We'll be away from my grandson Oakley for several weeks. And a day without seeing Oaks is like a day without sunshine for his granddad, JD.

Cruis'n - September 16, 2013

Just when you think things can't get any *better*, they do. I turned that phrase around because it reflects my mood as I sit on our ship cabin's veranda overlooking the exotic port of Dubrovnik, Croatia. We celebrated our thirty-eighth wedding anniversary last night with the bottle of champagne we won dancing; and the Bucket List adventure continues.

Taking a cruise is expensive, but investing in memories is priceless. Cruising is a unique way to travel because you take your hotel room with you as you travel to the next port while you sleep. Also you're spared the daily task of packing and unpacking, and all your meals are paid for. It's a real treat when Becky and I go out to a nice restaurant at home; but on a cruise, it's fine restaurant dining every night.

Our ship is home to 2000 guests and 800 crew members, but it's only half the size of an aircraft carrier with a complement of 5000 souls. And our floating hotel is far more luxurious than the Navy's and includes more food than you should eat, and complimentary room service if you desire. Nightly, we're entertained by Broadway class singers and dancers, Cirque du Soleil-like performers, piano bar vocalists, and classical violinists. There's always something to do, or you can just sit on the deck and people-watch or snooze. And shore excursions enable you to see the wonders of the world and experience different cultures. Years ago I considered becoming a cruise ship's doctor, but finally concluded it's good to travel, but even better to come home.

In the opinion of this temporary "travel writer," Venice, Italy is the most interesting city in the world. We spent two days ashore exploring the small twisted streets which traverse innumerable canals by graceful half-moon shaped bridges. Canals are the real *streets* of Venice, and give this floating city its unique charm. The city sits atop one hundred and seventeen islands all supported by pylons which are trying to save the city from sinking into the marsh. This seems to be a losing battle despite efforts of the Venetians because the city is sinking nine inches a year.

In Venice it's really odd to hear an ambulance and look up to see yellow Sea Ray-like boats rushing to the rescue. And rush hour on the choked canals of "Venezia" is strange with delivery barges, public transportation-boats and taxi-boats, amidst gondolas and the private boats of Venetians who pay for boat slip parking just as we pay for street parking.

Have you ever noticed how different your neighborhood looks when you walk rather than drive? The view from our Tennessee River is certainly different than from the banks. And no trip to Venice is complete without the view from one of its signature gondolas. When I was young and bumbling around Europe before medical school, I couldn't afford a gondola ride; this time I could. Becky admitted that she selected Roberto as our gondolier because he was "Italian-handsome." She chose wisely because our ride on the Grand Canal was made even more memorable by his musical Italian elocution.

I've always had wanderlust and I've traveled to a lot of places, but few as beautiful as Dubrovnik, Croatia or Kotor, Montenegro. These countries were formed by the Yugoslavian wars of the 1990s. You may recall names like Sarajevo, Bosnia or Kosovo, but these strange places become more real when you stand in Dubrovnik and see the city's scars from Serbian and Montenegrin shelling. The name Yugoslavia means "all the Slavs" yet there are other ethnic groups and religions in this tortured part of the world. With the death of the Soviet era dictator, Tito, they fell upon each and the rest is history.

I take no sides in these recent wars of nationalistic and ethnic cleansing because there are enough faults to go around. I see only the sad repetition of history. In 100 AD the Roman emperor Trajan conquered this same region and annihilated the country and people of Dacia. The only remnants are the modern people of Romania, whose Romanian is even more Latinized than other Romance languages.

Today Dubrovnik and Kotor are UNESCO cultural heritage sites and wondrous. Both have "old city" areas that date to the Middle Ages. From the winding and narrow streets you hear exotic music from radios and the strange language of people correcting their children and chatting as they hang their wash from their windows to dry in the Mediterranean sunshine. We scaled the walls of the old forts and walked everywhere taking pictures that we may never look at again, but it's what tourists do to help them remember places they'll probably never see again.

We Southerners have a reputation for being hospitable, but we were made similarly welcome in a cliff-side cafe above the Adriatic in Dubrovnik, and in an alfresco cafe in Kotor. Perhaps it's just easier to be hospitable in small towns as opposed to New York or Paris.

We've now rounded the corner in our journey, and the "CA Tour Group" is on the homeward stretch. We left Corfu, Greece today (the birthplace of Prince

Phillip) and sailed westward across the Ionian Sea. By the time you read this we'll have traversed the Strait of Messina and the boot of Italy, and will soon be in the Eternal City.

Rome, the capital of the Roman Empire, lasted a thousand years. Saint Augustine and the ancients thought the city was eternal. That perspective proved wrong when it was sacked by the Visigoths in the fourth century AD. Many have compared America to ancient Rome. I hope they're wrong.

Bellissimo - September 23, 2013

I am a Trinitarian at heart, and Becky maintains that I can find three choices for any situation. This is because I believe four choices are too many in most situations, and two are too few. I'm not a numerologist, but one choice is no choice at all, so you can see why I opt for three.

I conclude my travel trilogy this week, and perhaps I'll return to some dry-as-toast medical topic next week, but I make no promises. As I've said before, I write about what intrigues me at the moment.

My life has been blessed, and I thank The Master daily for Grace, a great marriage and reasonably good health. I was also blessed with good parents who taught me virtue and about patriotism. They enabled me to obtain a first class education, and they encouraged me to expand my horizons by seeing the world. Most of us remember the story of George Bailey in **It's a Wonderful Life**. George wanted to travel the world, but never did. I have seen the world, and I've also had a wonderful life.

Language intrigues me. We use words as tools to exchange detailed information with each other. The Tower of Babel is an ancient story where man became too prideful and attempted to build a tower (probably a ziggurat) to Heaven. The story continues as God thwarts those efforts by introducing various languages among the builders who were then unable to continue their Led Zeppelin-esque "Stairway to Heaven."

I've coordinated a half dozen medical mission trips to Guatemala in Central America. In the mountains we cared for descendants of the Mayans who still speak dialects of ancient Quiche. Do you remember the Star Trek character Warf? He is a fictional Klingon, and if you've heard his guttural sounding speech on TV with its abrupt and clipped cadence, replete with clicking sounds from the back of his throat, you get some sense of Quiche.

I was similarly flummoxed once riding a tram in Prague. Slavic languages are alien to a westerner's ear. I couldn't understand the stops when called by the Czech conductor despite the tram map in my hand. Romance languages like Spanish and French, whose roots are Roman, are easily recognizable – even if you don't understand what they're saying. I'm glad English is my native language, though I've been a student of English since first grade. English is an amalgam of many languages and I'm told it's a hard language to master. I guess that's true because the British, New Yorkers, and Southerners all have such a hard time understanding each other! And I won't mention the dialectical issues of Aussies or the brogue of my friends in Edinburgh, Scotland.

I had two somewhat selfish goals when I convinced Becky and our friends to accompany me on my "Bucket Trip". Our expectations were exceeded as we experienced the Dalmatian coast. Now, it's on to Rome and the last treasure on my list.

The great Renaissance sculpture Michelangelo is best known for his paintings of the Sistine Chapel. Included is the iconic **Creation of Adam** depicting God's life-giving touch reaching across space and time to bring life to the listless Adam. Michelangelo didn't want the project because he thought painting was an inferior art-form to sculpting. However, Pope Julius II *insisted*, ultimately making him an offer he couldn't refuse: the young upstart Raphael would be given the commission. So, Michelangelo relented and daily hoisted himself onto a scaffold one hundred feet above the floor of the Pope's new chapel for four years, completing his monumental work in 1512. To see this masterpiece cleaned of the soot and grime of centuries, releasing the master's color-filled palate, was a twenty-five year dream of mine now fulfilled.

Raphael was not to be denied because next door to the Chapel he painted his own masterpiece, **The School of Athens**. Years ago I served as a volunteer docent at the Knoxville Museum of Art guiding tours of the exhibits. I've often compared other works to these masterpiece frescoes of Michelangelo and Raphael whose visions and colors are now forever embedded within the Vatican's plaster walls.

Art is, I believe, unique to the beholder. Not everyone will be moved by Michelangelo's and Raphael's works, or by my passion. I do believe that as you learn about something, you appreciate it more. However, I also hold to the Count Basie theory, "If it sounds good it is," and if it's pleasing to the eye and gives you joy, it's likewise good.

Our guide for the day and new friend Nino showed us his city Rome, or as he says, "Roma" with his lyrical Italian that made me think of Roberto our gondolier in Venice. Rome is a city of five million with 600 churches and 300 fountains.

Ancient ruins mingle with modern life powered by Smart cars and scooters which seem to commix with pedestrians. As tourists we saw the Coliseum that once held 50,000 spectators for gladiatorial games, and the Circus Maximus where Charlton Heston, as the fictional Ben Hur, raced chariots before 250,000 cheering Romans. We saw the Forum, monuments and dozens of churches. It's not surprising that there are so many churches in Rome. After all, the great historian Will Durant once observed that "Christ conquered Caesar," it just took 300 years until the Emperor Constantine declared Christianity the official religion of the Roman Empire.

I'll end with kudos for Michelangelo and Raphael and an Italian adjective for Bernini's magnificent Trevi Fountain – BELLISSIMO!

The Test - February 24, 2011

By the time you read this I'll know the result of my test. Most of us have been sick enough to consult a doctor and go for an examination and tests. And we've all had the agony of waiting for these test results. I tell my patients that we have a system to contact them that same day if a test result is out of the acceptable range. This eases a patient's mind. I then emphasize that I will mail them a copy of their test results with an explanatory note. I believe this creates a partnership system of checks and balances between me and my patients. I tell them no test is *normal* until they hear from me; and they're encouraged to call me if they don't receive even normal results in two weeks.

When I was more involved in the training of young doctors I often challenged them with the notion that they would eventually suffer from many of the diseases of their patients. Not surprisingly these young doctors had trouble imagining chronic pain, and failing organs and faculties. I recall one intern who cocked his head slightly and furrowed his brow in a quizzical manner as he considered my observational wisdom. His mannerism made me think of my dog's reaction when he hears a strange noise and tilts his head back and forth trying to triangulate the sound. I kept this vision to myself and instead told him to reflect on what I'd said and to try and imagine things from a patient's perspective as he examined them. It's called empathy.

I now wait for my test result that will be a watershed event for my career, if not my life. Some people believe that our universe and each of us are nothing more than chance events. This perspective maintains that given enough time and opportunity you'd be reading this essay in the Knoxville Focus. A man named Boltzman purported to have calculated the probability that our universe would be as we now observe it due to chance. Boltzman found that it is very unlikely that we're a random collection of events – one chance in 10 with eighty zeros by Dr. B's calculus. It is certainly possible that everything is random and chance, but I find this so unlikely that I dismiss the notion of a random universe.

Others say that we are part of a reality that has design and purpose and a Designer. I have to admit that the purpose is often inscrutable to me, but my vision and knowledge are admittedly limited. There may be a middle position where the Designer intercedes in big events as I believe happened 2000 years ago, and the rest of the time we operate under the laws of physics, chemistry, neurobiology and freewill.

I'm reading Bobby Drinnon's book that chronicles his life story and his *gift*. Mr. Drinnon lives in Talbot, Tennessee, and is described by some as a psychic. He is certainly a Christian spiritualist. Many years ago, with prompting from friends and my skeptical scientist's hat firmly affixed atop my head, I went to see Mr. Drinnon. My conclusion of our meeting is that he is a person with extreme empathy which he describes as *intuitive awareness*. What if there are people who sense things on other planes or to a greater degree than others? After all, I believe each of us possesses intuition as a *sixth* sense in addition to our five senses. Our intuition is an amalgam of our other senses coupled with reason. Perhaps there are even more levels of awareness.

It may be risky or maudlin to tell the story of my illness and my test, but it's a story we all experience sooner or later. As a defense, I have to write about what's on my mind and in my heart at the moment. I've found that writing to fill an assignment reads like a greeting card; whereas writing from the heart is real and is as palpable as a swollen knee.

My readers know that I am a scientist, but one who has acquired a spiritual perspective as well. My vision is much broader now and much more complex. This other outlook is also a comfort and an assurance that doesn't lead to deception as some have argued. As I wait for my test result I have a sense of calm that I have to admit feels a bit surreal. I realize it could go either way for me. I've lived sixty wonderful years and I hope the journey continues. Time and the test will tell.

My doctor just called me with my test results! I'm OK, and I get to go on!!

I don't understand it, but Becky loves to pick blackberries. And since I love her, I'm often pressed into service this time of year. I do love eating blackberries, sometimes as I pick them, but don't tell my wife who wants the berries for pies. The trick is to not consume like the Coneheads of Saturday Night Live, and to save enough berries for blackberry jam to enjoy all winter long.

Most of the time berry picking is a solitary endeavor. Though the occasional, "Ouch" is heard from the adjoining brush, there's usually not a lot of banter. As I harvested the lush bounty of summer (and yes, ate my fill like an ole bear preparing for winter) my essay of the week came to me. You might find this strange, but it's really not, because our world is full of stories if you have "eyes to see."

Blackberries usually ripen around the Fourth of July in our area, but it's been warmer this year and they're coming in season now. And so as I participate in the harvest my mind wanders, until I'm pricked back to reality by the evolutionary survival advantage (thorns) nature afforded blackberry plants.

We are all solar powered. No, I'm not talking about the politically correct and not ready for prime time "Green Energy" imbroglio. I'm talking about stellar fusion of hydrogen that powers our sun and the stars of the universe. Imagine millions of nuclear bombs exploding every second, majestically balanced by the sun's gravitational collapse, and you have a picture of our sun. Now imagine the radiant energy of those explosions streaming across space to warm and power our earth. This same energy flows into the blackberries which I now pick. Actually, I'm consuming their stored solar energy.

As I worked my way through the patch I observed various stages of the fruit's development. Some berries receiving less light were still green and others were further along, moving through a beautiful red to the coveted succulent black. The colors made me think of checker boards and bruises.

Bruises!? Where's he going with this, you ask? If you've ever picked blackberries you know that it's virtually impossible to pick them and avoid pricking your fingers; that is unless you forage in a hybrid berry patch. A hemophiliac should not pick wild blackberries. No pain, no gain I say, as I scan the stains on my fingers and wonder how much is from berry juice or the drops of blood from pricks akin to diabetic testing.

We take the healing of injured parts for granted. With injury a majestic and intricate repair process is activated. First, tiny blood elements called *platelets* plug the hole caused by the blackberry thorn. Next, coagulation proteins coalesce and form a temporary patch over the platelet plug. Finally, our natural *repair workers* (white blood cells) show up with the equivalent of reconstruction blueprints, dry wall, spackling and paint. When the boo-boo is repaired, the healing process shuts down; if it doesn't and proceeds without control, cancer results. This whole process is organized and directed by chemicals called *cytokines* produced and released by the injured cells.

All of us have experienced a bruise. Imagine blood as red as an unripe blackberry escaping from a punctured blood vessel. Hopefully, the rupture is plugged, but the already extruded blood collects and eventually the red blood cells begin to breakdown, releasing their oxygen-carrying hemoglobin proteins. You've undoubtedly noticed that venous blood is a deeper maroon color because it has already given up some of the oxygen while coursing through capillary beds. As hemoglobin gives up its oxygen, the molecule changes shape and reflects light at a different wave length which we see as a different color. The same process occurs in a bruise as the pigments change and go through an evolution of colors. Blackberries transform from green to red to black. Bruises go from red to bluish-black and even to greenish and yellowish hues.

Our ability to see occurs on multiple levels. Is there more than what we perceive? Sometimes we get so wrapped up in ourselves we don't consider the perspective of others or see other realities around us. Have you ever watched ants? I don't think they operate by reason, but they have a reality just as we do.

I once imagined our solar system as an atom with the nucleus analogous to our sun. And swirling around the nucleus were planets instead of electrons. Could our solar system and others be a part of a leaf on some cosmic tree catching and storing light like blackberry bushes? I wonder what would happen if our cosmic berry was picked, or if we would even perceive pigment changes in our leaf in the fall of the year.

Poet laureate Robert Frost once observed that the snowy woods around his sleigh were "...lovely, dark and deep." The universe is also, and wondrous whether we perceive it or not. It extends from quasars to quarks and beyond, even to the throne of Creation and Creator.

67

A Life Well Lived - September 6, 2011

"He was a man, take him all in all, I shall not see his like again."
William Shakespeare, *Hamlet*

I lost a friend today, and it has really affected me. As a doctor of internal medicine and geriatrics who still sees patients in the hospital, I'm around sickness and death all the time. But, you're never prepared for the "call in the middle of the night" if it's your children, your parents or close friends.

David was a man's man and the patriarch of his family. He had worked his way to prominence in a major European company, had survived the long wait for coronary bypass surgery in the United Kingdom, and came through his surgery with flying colors three years ago. He wrote to me that he was back climbing mountains in the Scottish Highlands and feeling great, but suddenly dropped dead while working out in the gym. Like *Braveheart*, I'm sure he's in his kilts without *encumberments*, and piping bagpipes amidst the heavenly hosts. But all of us left behind are forever changed.

I seem to be going to more funerals these days as those in my cohort get older and *pass away*. I wonder if this softer phraseology is better than saying David died suddenly with what doctors call "sudden cardiac death." We, the living, tend to mince our words striving for political correctness and sensitivity when speaking of death. The black community uses the term "passing on" instead of away. I find this perspective closer to mine and a comfort. I wish I could be in Edinburgh for David's wake and funeral to support his family in their grief. Funerals are for the living, you know. David is already fine.

Several years ago I published my first novel and invited some friends to a book signing to celebrate this milestone with me. The gathering was held at my Church *down by the river*. Becky and I thought there'd be twenty-five to forty family members, close friends and church supporters. I was astounded to see the people who just kept coming and filled our riverside pavilion. They bought my book because they loved me; few had ever read a work of science fiction. It was a moving experience, and as I penned personal remarks and my signature in each book, I had the distinct vision of my own funeral, but with the unique opportunity to actually experience the support and affirmation of a job well done.

Everyone wants the approval of those they serve and love; you're especially blessed if this approval is for your life's work. One of the joys of being a doctor is the relationship you have with those you care for and advise over the years. But, it's also a two-edged sword. Doctors are peculiar because anytime one of their patients does badly, the immediate reaction is, "Oh no, what did I miss?" It's a bit like being a parent; when your child does well you beam and say, "Look what my child has done!" And when something goes badly you ask yourself, "How did I ruin this poor child?" Maybe we all have a bit of *Jewish mother* in us.

One night, years ago, I met my friend and patient in the emergency room with her husband; and she was desperately ill. As we worked to care for her she looked up and asked me, "Jim, am I going to die?" And she did, a short time later, virtually in my arms.

Most of life is not as poignant or dramatic as these stories. We could search for meaning in their untimely deaths or even debate the Teacher's philosophy in the third chapter of Ecclesiastes. A better perspective is one that honors life and those who have gone before us. I love the quote of a Jewish rabbi I read in a book once who said that all he wanted was to "live with a sense of wonder." I try to think of this each day as I awaken and I'm granted another day to savor and to serve.

At the US National Tennis Center a statue of the great American tennis player Arthur Ashe is inscribed with his life philosophy, "A job is the way to make a living; service is the way to make a life."

Well said, Mr. Ashe. His perspective should be the mantra of the living. We should go each day and do our best and our duty for God and country and all those we love and serve. This is the meaning of life and it honors the fallen.

The world is very complicated, and I can see why some folks just withdraw from the modern techy world. I'm proud of my mother who has not given up, and not only lives independently, but does email and even follows her family and friends on Face Book. It takes courage to be "out there" in the world of cyberspace. I'm still unsure of myself when I post on Face Book. Recently, Becky was surprised by comments after her inaugural Face Book post about our anniversary. One quipped, "Well, it's about time!" Mistakenly, Becky announced our nuptials, after thirty-eight years of marriage.

My sister-in-law finally converted to a smart phone after I shamed her while repairing the cover of her old flip-phone. Now, she not only makes phone calls, but she's able to check her email and text her family. I admit that I resisted texting, but finally concluded that I had to do so if I wanted to stay in touch with my kids. These 21st century philosophs are tech and social media savvy. Now, I find I'd rather receive a text with a pic than an email or a phone call. Trust me; texting is wonderful technology, and keeps my family connected across considerable distances. Oakley's parents can even keep up with the boy's activities as pictures pop up on their iPhones throughout the day.

Some say we've become a slave to our technology. I'll admit I've been guilty of whipping out my iPhone when something pops into my mind. Another advantage of the new technology is that I carry around fewer scraps of paper with notes. Now, when I want to know something I just Google it, and go the reference desk of the worldwide web library. For an inquisitive guy the Net is an irresistible siren's song. However, a word of caution, a Google search should not interrupt dinner conversation!

The biggest problem with all this technology is keeping it working. My first car was a used Ford Mustang. In those days boys worked on cars. I'm no mechanic, but I replaced the water pump on my "rod", did all the maintenance work, and even adjusted the timing belt and set points on the distributor before modern electronic ignition technology. Have you looked under the hood of a car lately? There's no room to spare as in olden days. We recently bought a hybrid and there is not only a standard engine under the hood, but an electric one as well. And the battery is in the trunk! What's a good ole boy to do?

Recently, my computer's hard drive began to fail and I was forced to buy a new laptop to write these essays and to interact with my concierge patients. After considering my needs and the options, I selected a new machine and that's when the fight began. I have a basic knowledge of how cars work. But computers are much more mysterious than a car. Perhaps it's because computers work on quantum mechanic principles which no one really understands. None the less, these tools work and are a necessary component of 21st century life. The problem is that computers and their software applications are complicated, and when something goes wrong you need an expert.

Foolishly, I assumed that the anti-virus protection that I purchase through my home internet server would transfer to my new computer automatically as so many other programs do. It did not this time and I was almost immediately invaded and overrun by malware. I needed what the street calls a "geek" – someone to clean up my computer mess. My anti-virus company fortunately provided Michael. This computer "parson" listened to my confession and then assumed control of my computer.

Jessica Tandy won an Oscar for her role in the movie **Driving Miss Daisy**. It's a beautiful story about an elderly southern matron and her trusted black chauffeur. The haughty Miss Daisy finally comes to grips with her prejudice. In some respects I felt as out of control as Miss Daisy when Michael took remote control of my computer and drove me around the internet. I marveled as Michael manipulated my computer to isolate the problems, orchestrate the remedy, and heal my broken machine. When it was all over, I heartily thanked him for the cure. I suspect my gratitude was comparable to a patient who has been healed by a skilled physician.

Yes, the world is complicated, but I'm not sure our complexity makes us any happier or better. Case in point, have you heard of ICD-10? Well, this government medical coding mandate is coming and will cause even more upheaval than Obama-care. Doctors and hospitals use diagnostic codes for various conditions. An example is 250.00 for adult type 2 diabetes. These codes were created decades ago for description of diseases, but are now used for billing purposes. The new system will replace ICD-9 and increase the number of disease codes from 17,000 to 155,000 descriptors, and will destroy what is left of our medical system. The implementation of this system will be very expensive with cost estimates of $30,000 per physician and an extra hour each day to properly code the patient's care. Furthermore, coding confusion will delay payments, sometimes for months leading to bankruptcy of the few small office practices that are left. So, why do we need codes for "drowning associated with one's water skis catching fire" or "suicide by jellyfish envenomation"? I'm not making this up, folks. These are real ICD-10 codes.

It is apparent to me that Barney Fife is now running virtually every area of our government, and we are in trouble. I happen to believe that medical care is not this complicated, and I believe we need to again embrace "care" of patients rather than following more mandated protocols (metrics) from central command in Washington. We may have one last chance to reverse the destruction. We'll see this November.

I literally jumped when the musical alarm went off, blaring, ♫ *She'll be coming around the mountain when she comes...!*

"What's going on?" I asked the hospital nurses who seemed oblivious to the irritating song which I've always disliked.

"It's a new regulation, Dr. Ferguson. All patients who are judged to be at risk of falling have to be on an alert monitor and this song was judged by plant engineering as being so irritating that it wouldn't be ignored. We even tried to change the melody and the hospital's engineer came and changed it back."

I had just arrived on the floor to make rounds on patients who had the unfortunate pleasure of being hospitalized on a Saturday. At that moment another alarm and stanza of *Oh Suzanna* erupted from another patient's room just down the hall.

"You've got to be kidding," I remarked. "Not only is that song loud, but obnoxious. How will patients get any rest if the darn thing goes off whenever they roll over? And the noise will drive all of you crazy and me as well."

They all shrugged their shoulders and reminded me that government regulations now prevent the use of the "*seat belts,*" formerly known as Posey restraints and were used to keep confused and frail patients from getting up without assistance and falling. There aren't enough sitters (or resources) to stay with so many patients twenty-four hours a day.

I flinched again as another alarm went off. "No, we're not kidding, Dr. Ferguson. We had seventeen patients on our floor last night and ten of them had the government mandated alarms."

I picked up my charts and went into my next patient's room. I found her sitting in a chair crying. I had admitted her the evening before with atrial fibrillation and heart failure. This distinguished lady had just come from her weekly appointment to the beauty shop and hadn't planned to be hospitalized. I couldn't help but notice the football helmet without a face guard she sported which was crushing yesterday's coiffure.

"Mrs. Jones, why are you wearing a helmet on your head?" I asked.

"They made me put it on," she sniffled, "because I'm on Coumadin and they say it's to protect my head if I fall down." I thought to myself that at least the hated song wasn't blaring. I asked her if she wanted to wear that helmet and she assured me to the contrary with a vigorous shake of her head. I said to her, "Well take the dang thing off and throw it in the floor." And she did so with relish and a smile.

Folks, this is what happens in a nanny state where thinking is replaced by protocols mandated by government bureaucrats, developed by central committees and guided by legal opinion. Don't get me wrong, as a geriatrician I know that sick or impaired patients need our protection, but the policies our hospital is forced to implement are ludicrous. People do fall down and they need our care, but we've replaced logic with protocols and insist that professional nurses function as drones and follow the policies of central command.

As I was lamenting the new policies with a neurosurgical colleague we got into a discussion regarding problem solving. He quoted a number of recent neurological studies which showed older doctors solve complex problems quicker than younger ones. These same studies did show that older docs were less efficient in multi-tasking, but they were still able to *cut to the chase* quicker and more efficiently. Perhaps this relates to what is known as *fuzzy logic*. Computers can crunch data at a speed of one hundred and eighty-six thousand miles a second (the speed of light). Neurons in our brains conduct electrochemical impulses at a maximum of 100 meters (about one hundred yards) a second. And yet the 100 billion brain cells we have between our ears, each with hundreds if not thousands of interconnections, work collectively to produce thinking humans. No machine comes close to our brain, especially if we get to use it to solve problems. This ability to think logically is what makes our species unique and conferred to our ancestors a survival edge.

We must never relegate our uniqueness to the whims of the State, no matter how well intentioned, or we risk losing our freedom to think if not our humanity.

I like to read several books at a time rather than reading one cover to cover. In one of my two weekly book groups we're reading *Miracles* by C. S. Lewis. By definition a miracle is a phenomenon that has no rational or scientific explanation. And herein is the conundrum according to Lewis. How can an event that defies human reason or measurement be explained? And yet most of us have experienced things that are seemingly beyond our understanding or definition.

Some years ago a patient came to me for advice and as I discussed her medical issues with her she suddenly stopped me and asked about my grandmothers. I was a bit puzzled by her tangential question, but I replied that both my grandmothers were dead. My patient encouraged me to continue. I told her one grandmother was your Norman Rockwell *prototypical* grandmother, and the other was not. I'm embarrassed to say so, but within our family the latter was known as *mean granny*. This was of course covert and undoubtedly unfair, but nonetheless was the family's moniker. A boy's memory is strangely influenced, but as an example one year my brothers and I received Christmas gifts of "soap on a rope."

As I sheepishly related these anecdotes to my patient, who described herself as *spiritually sensitive*, she then informed me with an earnest face that my departed grandmother was standing behind me and wanted to say that she was sorry.

You can imagine my surprise and perhaps some unease to hear that behind me was my "mean granny's" specter. I managed to keep my cool and ventured a look over my left shoulder, but I could see nothing. I told my patient that I wasn't angry with my grandmother and that apologies weren't necessary, but if accepting her apology made her feel better, then her apology was accepted.

A strict rationalist might say that I fed my patient's delusions, but I can say that she was otherwise completely sane. A philosophic definition of the Natural world might be "what we perceive with our five senses." However, our preconceived notions of reality color the interpretation of our senses. A man named Rene Descartes felt that his reason was being influenced by his senses. So, he isolated himself in a darkened, quiet room and finally concluded, "Cogito ergo sum." (I think therefore I am.)

The point of this digression is that none of us is without bias. Scientists tell us of the sub-atomic world of zooming particles which don't obey the laws of Newtonian physics. We know of these particles only because their tracks have been recorded in cloud chambers designed to measure them as they pop into and out of our Universe. But are they real if we've never seen them?

A wise physician once told me that "Doctors often treat, sometimes cure, but should always care." I believe he was right. Sometimes we can't save our patients from the inevitable. Some years ago a patient of mine suffered a brain hemorrhage and was on a ventilator. The family and I finally concluded that he could not recover and the machine that tethered him to this reality should be stopped. It is said that a human can fast for weeks or months before dying. Science also says that you will die in a week or so if deprived of water. However, the brain and the heart will stop in minutes if they are deprived of circulating oxygen.

His family tearfully said goodbye to him and left the nurse and me to turn off the machine and inform them when their father had "passed away." After turning off the ventilator, we watched the heart monitor and waited and waited. Five minutes went by, then ten, then twelve... All the while the nurse and I kept the vigil, becoming increasingly incredulous. Thirteen minutes, fourteen minutes and the situation became eerie. Suddenly, at fifteen minutes my patient raised his arms as if reaching for something above his bed. This lasted for only a few moments and then his arms fell to his sides and his heart monitor fell silent.

I admit that I have a scientific bias. As an internist I search for explanations of symptoms and the cause of disease. I could explain the spiritualist's observations as quirky, and the man's levitation to a condition called decerebrate posturing. But can I be sure that I'm not prejudiced by my a priori scientific notion of reality?

An American philosopher (and atheist) named William James said in so many words that if there are two divergent perspectives, and there are no incontrovertible proofs that either is right or wrong, then a rational person is free to choose which ever perspective works best for him.

I might take issue with James' *pragmatism* that implies an either/or choice. I am a scientist, but I have a spiritual perspective as well. As a scientist I keep my eyes open on the natural world. And I keep my heart open to the directives of the Spirit as well.

Priorities change as we get older. I sense that several of you are already nodding your heads knowingly. And I have to admit that my attitude about keeping up with the most recent advances in internal medicine seems less important to me now than when I first became a doctor in 1975. I still read seven medical journals regularly, keep up with required CME (continuing medical education) and go to medical seminars, but I've come to realize that the newest information does not always stand the test of time. *Change* doesn't always work out for the best. When I began my practice I lived and breathed internal medicine, but now I'm more drawn to the momentous events taking place in our world and our country. So again, I write about what's on my heart and mind; forgive me if you were in the mood for a medical tutorial.

How do we collect information and make decisions? That seems obvious, but internists think about *why* things happen. All of us use our eyes, ears, nose, touch and occasionally our taste buds to measure the world before sending the information to our brains to sort out. Doctors collect data from their patients, evaluating history and physical findings. Then doctors compare the situation against normal physiology and their knowledge of disease. We then formulate a hypothesis and often test these hunches with X-Rays and lab work. But is that all there is? Have you ever *felt* something was wrong on an instinctual or "gut level?" Men have learned to trust this visceral equivalent of a "woman's intuition."

I called upon my gut feelings recently as we flew home from a family vacation in Alaska. On boarding the plane in Seattle I was called to help a fifty year old man who was having chest pain, shortness of breath and was pale, sweaty and anxious. He told me that he was a businessman, traveling all over the world by airplane. He also told me his father had died of a heart attack in his fifties.

I told the flight attendants that this man should not take a long cross-country flight, but should go to the hospital and be evaluated. Instead, the EMTs (Emergency Medical Technicians) were called onto the plane to assess the man. They couldn't find anything <u>measurably</u> wrong with him. Furthermore, he refused to go to the hospital and be properly evaluated.

"Perhaps I'm over reacting," I thought. But, if there is nothing medically wrong with the man, why is he so nervous? And why is he clutching his leather mail satchel across his chest, and continuously rocking back and forth? I kept looking back at "my patient" as our plane taxied down the runway. Intermittently, he would turn and look out his bulkhead window, but most of the time he just sat there with his eyes closed and head bobbing. Is there another explanation for this Jordanian man's anxiety?

As we readied ourselves for take-off, my wife and I continued discussing our suspicions, and finally concluded the man might be a terrorist. And if he was and detonated his satchel at 35,000 feet over the Rockies in the middle of the night, we would all die. At the very least I felt this man was medically unstable and may be suffering from angina. The thought of an in-flight heart attack and resuscitation was something I didn't want to face.

My wife and I have lived a blessed life and have told ourselves many times that if it's our time to go, it's been a good run. However, my daughter was sitting between us and my niece was just behind us. These young folks were just beginning their lives and inaction that endangered them was unacceptable to my wife and me. For the first time in our lives we pushed the emergency button telling the stewardess we wanted off the airplane.

We aborted the takeoff, and forced the plane to return to the gate where our family marched off the airplane. Yes, we took bold action without knowing all the facts, because I thought this man's health might be in danger, and all of our lives perhaps depended upon my willingness to trust my instincts. Finally, the pilot ordered the man off the plane and we re-boarded and continued our journey home. Later, other passengers and the flight attendants thanked us repeatedly for insisting that the man be removed from the plane to get help.

You may not realize that a passenger may leave a plane if he feels afraid to fly or uncomfortable with decisions of the flight crew. We were taking the last plane out of Seattle on July 4th and flying to Obama's Chicago. I disagreed with the man's refusal to get proper medical care, and I felt very uncomfortable with the Captain's initial refusal to order the man off the plane. The Captain finally relented.

It seems to me that the issue of personal responsibility is now the major focus in our country. Are we content to trade our freedoms of choice, and their consequences, for the perceived safety and security of the State? I could have depended on the flight attendants and the Captain of the airplane to take care of my family. But, they refused to act prudently. And as I sat there with everyone I love, the situation just didn't feel right medically and otherwise.

What would you have done? Would you have stepped out in faith or played it politically correct? Do you believe that the State can or will take care of you? Are you willing to write or call your Congressmen and Senators and tell them what you think of the momentous issues facing our country?

There is another aspect of this story that has never been told. As my family de-boarded the airplane and reentered the now semi-dark concourse, I stopped to explain the situation to the perplexed gate agent. It was then that we noticed a woman standing in the shadows thirty feet from my huddled family. She wore the traditional Muslim hijab. My wife noted she wore an airport identity badge, but made no attempt to interact with anyone. In fact, as the man was subsequently escorted from the plane by our gate agent, she disappeared into the empty concourse.

I felt sorry for the man who was removed from the flight, and sat on the other side of the concourse alone awaiting help. I don't know what happened to him because my family voted to re-board the plane and continue our journey. The vote was five to four. The rest of the story is anti-climactic. We did enjoy the complimentary champagne provided by the stewardesses. They all agreed the man needed medical evaluation.

In the next few days Becky contacted the airline and was stonewalled, though they did send us two complimentary vouchers for future air flights. We also spoke with the anti-terrorism expert Steve Emerson of the Investigative Project. After hearing our story, he told us we did the right thing, though we will never know if we aborted a terrorist attack.

Perhaps it is time to stand up for family, neighbors and country. We cannot afford to be uninformed, play it safe with our silence, or be distracted by our latest cholesterol reading while "Rome burns."

Several weeks ago I did a column on cardiovascular circulation. I used the metaphor of dump trucks in describing red blood cells which are "loaded" with oxygen and pumped around to the organs and tissues. We take for granted that we'll have enough red blood cells to carry enough oxygen to meet our needs, but unfortunately "[Stuff] happens," as Forrest Gump once said. Frequently, I'm called upon to evaluate and treat *anemia*, defined as a deficiency of red blood cells.

Humans make a protein called *globin* which is complexed with iron *heme* and incorporated into red blood cells as hemoglobin. The hemoglobin molecule "holds" the oxygen as it is carried to our organs in the blood stream. Imagine a dump truck carrying concrete to a construction site that discharges its load on arrival. How fascinating is the similarity between the oxygen carrying hemoglobin and the plant molecule chlorophyll. The latter takes the sun's energy, uses the carbon dioxide we exhale, and makes plant leaves and flowers, all the while "exhaling" oxygen back into the atmosphere. And where does iron come from that is so necessary to make this crucial molecule for our red blood cells? Iron is the end product (the ashes) of stellar fusion, the process that powers the sun. As Carl Sagan once said, "We are star stuff."

Anemia can occur from many causes, but I want to focus on one of the most common of human conditions, *iron deficient anemia*. It is estimated that 3.5 billion people have iron deficiency, and iron deficiency is the most common cause of anemia in the United States, affecting some 3 million women. Though necessary for health, only about 10% of dietary or supplemental iron is normally absorbed. Consequently, we can readily become iron deficient and anemic due to a poor or quirky diet, intestinal bleeding, serious medical illnesses, menstruation and pregnancy, and occasionally from mal-absorption due to medications or even tea.

Patients frequently complain of fatigue and my job is to discover the cause – and I believe there is always a cause whether science has a sufficient lens to see it. Many years ago I was taught that fatigue with a near normal blood count wasn't due to iron deficient anemia. Well, that was wrong, because we now understand that iron is critical for the growth of all cells and facilitates chemical reactions in our body. And since our body runs on chemistry, it's obvious that we might suffer if the reactions occur sluggishly. There may be something to the old *Geritol* ads that hawked the treatment of "iron poor blood."

Years ago I published a scientific paper on iron deficient anemia presenting with a condition called *pica*. The word derives from the Latin word for the magpie, a beautiful bird that nonetheless will eat almost anything. My patients hesitantly told me that they had developed peculiar cravings for dirt, ice, carrots and even laundry starch! It turns out that these cravings go away when iron deficiency is diagnosed and treated. I believe that the cravings associated with pregnancy are a form of pica and occur as vital iron stores are transferred to the baby, allowing the child to grow and make its own red blood cells. Have any of you ladies developed a peculiar craving for crunchy pickles during pregnancy or sent your husband out for other strange midnight food requests?

Perhaps there is balance in nature beyond our present understanding. Humans have a poor ability to absorb iron, but also an inability to rid ourselves of excess iron that can cause damage to the liver and other organs in certain genetic syndromes like Hemochromatosis. Iron overload can also occur in repeated transfusions with certain congenital blood disorders like Thalassemia. The usual challenge is to get enough iron and best accomplished by eating red meat and liver – I can't stand the thought of the latter having once worked in a VA hospital. Or you can take multivitamins with iron with your doctor's advice.

The main point is that there is a reason for your fatigue. Make sure it isn't due to a common and treatable problem like iron deficiency anemia. That would be poor stewardship. Like the Army mantra, we doctors want you to "be all you can be!"

I keep coming back to the topics that resonate with me and my patients. A couple came to see me recently because of his memory issues and declining function. *Mrs. Jones* described instances of her husband getting lost, forgetting the names of his children and even the kid's recent visit. During the interview, I observed my uncharacteristically quiet patient and silently made the unpleasant diagnosis.

About a year ago I wrote about the aggravating forgetfulness that occurs as we age and what distinguishes normal aging from what we doctors call *dementia*. There are certain dread words that cause such anxiety doctors try to avoid their usage until one is certain of the diagnosis. An example is the "C" word, cancer; another is Alzheimer's disease.

It might surprise you to learn that the original description by Dr. Alzheimer of the dementia that bears his name occurred in "pre-senile" patients. The implication being that older patients are expected to lose their memory and cognitive abilities. It is true that this dreaded condition increases with age (one in three after age eighty-five years old); it is not an inevitable outcome even in centenarians.

So why do some people get dementia, others vascular disease, and others cancer, lupus, or even COPD (chronic obstructive lung disease)? Recently, I was shocked to discover that a basic mechanism may be at work in all of these diverse maladies, even lung disease so often attributed to smoking. It turns out that genetic susceptibilities contribute to aberrant processing of environmental agents which results in inflammatory damage in diverse organs of the body. Two articles in the *New England Journal of Medicine* presented me a compelling theory why some people can smoke two packs of Camels a day and never get lung disease, and why some people become demented while others do not.

The Human Genome Project is a milestone of human technology. We now have a blue print of the human genome (DNA sequence). Someday doctors will be able to compare a patient's genome to the standard human DNA sequence and tell whether a patient has a disease susceptibility or whether a disease is inevitable. In the case of Huntington's disease, which caused dementia and death in Woody Guthrie, we can already do this. Unfortunately, it's not so simple in other diseases which may be due to multiple genetic anomalies or exposure to toxic agents like smoke. Do you remember the *nature vs. nurture* concept discussed some weeks ago? Well, it's some of both in most diseases.

This brings me back to the brain – that organ of 10 billion interconnected neurons – which makes humans, as far as we know, unique. Did you know that the back of your brain is the visual area? Did you realize that above your ears is where memories are stored in the brain? And behind your forehead is the frontal cortex of the brain, the area most important for our humanness and rational thought. Compare the same forehead area on your dog and then your cat. Ours is comparatively larger. You can begin to see why humans can think abstractly, consider our purpose in the Universe, conceive of time and have a sense of the Ideal, even its antithesis. The frontal area is damaged in Alzheimer's disease and causes us to lose aspects of our humanity and uniqueness.

Some anthropologists have argued that our forebrain developed when our ancestors began to stand upright on their hind legs in order to see above the tall grasses of the Serengeti Plain of Africa. Walking on hind legs perhaps freed up the arms of our ancestors and promoted the development of an opposable thumb and an enlarging motor area of the brain to control fine movement. Neuroanatomists have mapped the structural representation of our body in an area of the brain we identify as the motor strip. The area's name is derived from the Latin word *homunculus* – the little man – and is the area where the movement of my fingers across this keyboard originates.

We humans may be unique in the Universe, but what a waste of space! I like to think that the wondrous force of creation continues across space and time. Sometimes, it's just hard for a *little man* to comprehend the Creator's majesty.

I often ask my patients what they're reading when they come to see me, and I notice the books of friends when I'm in their homes. Most of us appreciate the recommendation of a good movie. Sharing the common experience of a good book or movie, a beautiful sunset or piece of music, or a memory brings us joy.

You can learn a lot about people and their culture if you observe their environment. When I travel I make it a point to browse the local market in addition to just watching people or taking in the sights. We used to do foreign mission work in Guatemala, and as we approached a village I frequently challenged my medical team to observe a village's farm animals and to notice if there were any cats or dogs. Ferguson's measure of a community's poverty and health is predicted by scarcity and condition of domestic animals. Though I have witnessed abject poverty in Haiti, it was in the mountains of Guatemala that I first observed *ribs on a pig* and understood poverty.

Becky and I recently spent the weekend with friends in their Smokey Mountain home. At four thousand feet it snows a lot in February and makes you appreciate the warmth of a fire and time to just sit, talk or read quietly, occasionally looking up to watch snow fall and coat the forest evergreens. We didn't miss the TV at all.

Some might find it unusual that I like to read several books at a time. It's quirky, but I've never had a problem catching up with plot even months later. As I browsed Mary's mountain library for a new book, I found one that had been recommended to me years ago, but I had never read. **The Tipping Point** is the first book by Malcolm Gladwell and describes "how little things can make a big difference." It is a fascinating book about human nature.

I'm a science fiction fan and remember Mr. Spock from the Star Trek series frequently using the word-phrase, "Fascinating!" I can identify with this notion because I find so many things fascinating. One of my many observations (which my partners refer to as Ferg-isms) is that you are old if things no longer fascinate you. If you're still searching for the medical perspective in this essay, you'll have to wait a bit. Perhaps anticipation will make the surprise segue better.

I met a miracle on the mountain. Some years ago a terrible industrial accident occurred at a foundry in Indiana. My friend's brother-in-law was literally burned to the bone when a forge of molten steel exploded. When I first heard of this injury I remember thinking that this was surely a mortal wound, and everyone thought he would die. But he didn't, and there he sat across the dinner table from me. Miraculously, I could hardly see the scars of his injuries. His ordeal was terrible, but I marvel at his recovery which seems to defy the notion of mortality.

I've heard it said that God will take you home when He gets you right. I've joked with patients who have come through seemingly impossible situations telling them "You must be here for a reason, Mrs. Jones, and be thankful God sent you back to me for remedial work!"

Most of us have experienced sunburn that results from the Sun's ultraviolet radiation. The red and sensitive skin is more apparent on Caucasians, but can occur in anyone and a burn of this extent is classified as a first degree burn. If the burn penetrates deeper into the skin and produces blisters, we doctors call this a second degree burn. I remember being put in charge of my younger brother at the beach one year while my Mom took my other brother to the doctor. I didn't listen to her about hats and sitting under the pool's umbrella, and sunscreen quickly washes off the body of a boy in the pool. I have personal knowledge of both first and second degree sunburns. In fact, my poor nose continues to reap the wages of youthful sun-sins.

Our skin is divided into three layers. The deepest layer is called the hypodermis and contains fat which helps to insulate us, provides padding and makes our ladies especially fetching. The next deepest layer is called the dermis and contains structural proteins (collagen and elastin), nerves, and blood vessels. As we age our skin loses elasticity as these skin proteins lose their flexibility. The dermal layer also helps regulate temperature by dilation and constriction of blood vessels. These blood vessels also nurture the most superficial layer of the skin called the epidermis. This outer layer keeps us from losing body water enabling us to live on land rather than being confined to the sea like our ancestors. And as we sweat through specialized pores in this layer our bodies are cooled by evaporation. Finally, you should never underestimate the value of epidermal appendages like fingernails or a luxurious head of hair!

If a burn extends through the epidermis and deeply into the dermis the skin cannot regenerate because the basal growth cells and their supporting blood vessels have been destroyed. In these settings skin grafting is necessary. You might picture this as analogous to putting sod on a barren yard. Harvested skin from unburned areas is often used to cover areas of a third degree burn. However, sometimes there isn't enough healthy skin available and artificial and animal tissues are used as temporary measures to close the holes and lessen massive fluid loss and limit invasive infection.

We are fortunate to have my new friend still with us. His courage (and his wife's) inspires me, and makes me reconsider the notion of a mortal wound. Medical science has certainly pushed back the notion of the impossible. But, what will happen when the money runs out and Obama's Panel says, "No mas"?

I probably live too much in "the world of cares." I'm sure I'd be happier if I were oblivious to the political war that is tearing our country apart. However, I've never been called to stand watch with an M-16 or fight in a foreign war in 120 degree heat. So, I look upon my engagement in politics (defined as the affairs of governance) as my *tour of duty*. I've been blessed to be an American, and now I have a duty to "speak the truth in love," at least until I'm silenced. Pericles, the great statesman of the ancient Athenian city-state, said that "people who say they're minding their own business and avoiding politics actually have no business here at all."

As I headed home dodging traffic on Alcoa Highway, a bumper sticker on a Prius caught my eye. Next to the Obama/Biden sticker was a second one that proclaimed, "I never used my civil liberties, anyway." As I drove past I glanced at the two women driving home just like me, and I wondered if they see the same country that I do. In a book I just finished the author observed that the United States has never been occupied by a foreign invader. Perhaps we have, if a majority of my countrymen do not ascribe to the ideals of the Constitution and think the rule of law which defines a republic is foolish.

There's much discussion lately regarding President Obama's comment that anyone's personal achievement only occurs within the framework of the government. This argument is fallacious yet continues to be proffered by the progressive Senator from Massachusetts and possible presidential candidate, Elizabeth Warren. Do you believe Bill Gates' genius only occurred because his parents afforded him space in their garage? Did this allow his creativity to blossom? By Obama's and Warren's reasoning, my hard work and sacrifice to get into medical school and graduate was only possible because of the State of Tennessee. I appreciate the sacrifice of men like my Dad who fought in the Second World War preserving my freedom and opportunities, but Obama's argument would make everyone a dependent and a slave of the state.

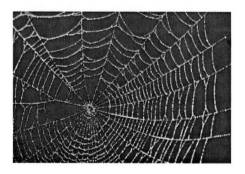

I'm reading a book called **The American Soul** by Jacob Needleman. The professor's study of Thomas Jefferson, Ben Franklin and George Washington reveals a common desire of these men to better themselves, not for the praise of other men, but to become better persons. The Master himself had similar advice to his followers two thousand years ago as chronicled in Matthew 6:5. I believe the desire to achieve comes from within, not from the state.

Studying the Founders has made me consider curiosity and why I want to know things just for the sheer joy of understanding. I don't know where this desire came from. I don't believe it was with me in grammar school or even high school that I remember.

I believe the joy of learning surfaced sometime in college, and it still burns brightly today. The ancient Greeks referred to this burning desire to know as "gnosis," from which we get the word knowledge. It pleases me to think I have something in common with the Founders of our country.

What happens if we lose the desire to help ourselves and expect others to pay for our upkeep and well-being? What if your own desires numb you to the feelings of others? In his book **Mere Christianity**, C. S. Lewis says that we are born with a conscience. He says that we act because we have a sense we "ought" to do so. Do you believe in right or that something is wrong? The sense of right seems to have been lost in Washington where politicians work in their own self-interest or party's rather than for the people or the country. The false idols of power and prestige are strong aphrodisiacs.

Even though our country is at war, I still see beauty and the reflection of the Creator in the world around me and in the gossamer webs of spiders. If distracted by the perverse media you might overlook the millions of spider webs around you, even though they're clearly visible in the early morning sunlight as it reflects on the dew coated webs. We need spiders because without them our world would be quickly overrun by insects. I think of spider webs as island universes amidst the expanse of the field around them. Each spider and its web is separated from the others, at least until we humans make the connection that we are all a part of the whole.

John Donne wrote that *"no man is an island"* in his Meditation XVII. I have to practice that perspective these days because of the political war swirling around me, and because in the world of electronic medical records I am forced to use, though there is no key stroke for **caring**.

We can't let ourselves become isolated or disengaged, nor can we give up and compromise our sense of what's right. The comic Groucho Marx once quipped,

"These are my principles; if you don't like them I have others." I can't do that. I can't go along to get along.

So where is the balance struck? A paraphrase of John Wesley's admonition has become my daily mantra. He said, "Do all you can, wherever you can, with everyone you can, as long as you ever can." Good marching orders for a citizen soldier in the midst of a civil war.

"Reality is always more than what we see."
Edmund Burke

The Universe is more wondrous than any of us can imagine. In recent weeks I've been talking about *seeing* and different levels of perception. In college I remember contemplating the limits of the Universe, from galaxies to the quantum realm. Now, science has extended that vision from quasars to quarks. Some years ago I was amazed when I first saw an electron microscopic picture of an atom which we were taught was the basic building block of all matter including trees and Fergusons. The word atom is of ancient Greek origin. Democritus imagined this basic building block of matter which he posited could not be split into smaller parts. Atom literally means unable to be cut. We know that atoms are comprised of protons, neutrons and electrons, and these protons and neutrons are made up of quarks, and some have imagined quarks as vibrating two-dimensional *strings* of energy. Maybe it goes on forever with ever-smaller fundamental parts.

In a similar manner we now see the Cosmos as vast and extending toward the limits of human imagination, and perhaps beyond. Imagine riding on the fastest spaceship ever constructed by humans toward the nearest star to our own sun. Alpha Centuri is only four light years away and yet it would take our hypothetical astronaut 70,000 years to get there with our current technology. Humbling, isn't it? Especially when you consider that the distant edge of the Universe is 13.5 billion light years away, and the Universe is still expanding ever faster into what, we don't know.

It is an allusion that our bodies are symmetrical and balanced as the Universe appears to be. I read a story once where scientists took digital pictures of people's faces. The researchers then digitally removed one half of the facial image, duplicated the remaining half, flipped it, and then put the facial image back together. Friends of the subjects were shown the reconstructed images and they couldn't recognize the person.

Most of us are not ambidextrous and recognize that one hand is dominant and one arm stronger as a result. I realize that my left eye is weaker than the other, and obviously this was the reason I couldn't pick up the spin of a curve ball well enough to become a major league baseball player. It wasn't my fault after all!

Many of us gravitate to certain careers that some believe is related to the so-called left or right brain dominance. It appears that the left side of your brain is oriented more to math and logic, whereas the right is preferential to the arts and esthetics. We certainly use both halves of our brains. There is evidence that genius may be associated with more highly developed *neural connections* in the corpus callosum that integrate the two halves. Congresswoman Gabby Gifford's speech center in the left side of her brain was damaged by the attack in Tucson Arizona. She is being trained to speak again through music therapy utilizing the undamaged right side of her brain.

I once had a patient whose brain was injured by a stroke within the deeper areas of his brain that integrated movement. As a result one of his arms was subject to sudden spasmodic jerks. Most of the time, Mr. Jones looked perfectly symmetrical and balanced. The problem arose when he and his wife decided to fly to the west coast and visit relatives. Apparently, the man in the seat next to Mr. Jones took umbrage at the repeated jabs in his side. Enough was enough when the meal tray arrived and was knocked into the man's lap; and that's when the fight began.

John Donne wrote that *"no man is an island"* in his Meditation XII. I have to practice that perspective these days because of the political war swirling around me and because in the mandated world of electronic medical records there is no keystroke for **caring**.

I hope that Thomas Paine will not be offended as I paraphrase his immortal words, "These are the times that try men's [waistbands]." The Thanksgiving cornucopia is past, but the Holiday Season has just begun, and the pounds must be addressed if we are to button slacks and zip our dresses.

My patient declared, "Doc, I'm on the 'Paleo Diet'." Fortunately, my Medicalese saved me from appearing totally flummoxed. When you go to medical school you learn a new language, the language of science derived from Latin and Greek root words. In addition to text books, I purchased Stedman's Medical Dictionary which was three and half inches thick. At first I looked up a lot of words as I studied, but as time went by fewer and fewer words stumped me. I actually looked up a word last summer and noticed the dust on the cover of my old dictionary. Calling upon my Latin I managed to reply, "Paleo means old, so I guess you're on a caveman's diet."

"You're right, Doc," and I could tell he was impressed that I knew about this latest craze. His "caveman" diet was based on what our hunter-gatherer ancestors were believed to have eaten. Their diet was meat, berries, nuts, whole grains and some plant vegetables. Our processed flour and sugar weren't yet invented and salt was scarce. I can understand the logic of this diet, but there is little science to support it. Had I been argumentative I might have pointed out the life expectancy was twenty-five years at the end of the last ice age (about 12,000 years ago). And a man five-foot-tall was a giant then.

There are many reasons why humans now live longer and grow taller than at any time in history. These include clean water, antibiotics, vaccinations, but also safe and better food that is also more plentiful. In fact, the food and drug regulatory agency (FDA) began in 1906 after Upton Sinclair published his sensational novel **The Jungle**, depicting the deplorable conditions in Chicago's meat industry.

We now have more processed food in our diets, and it is tempting to conclude that altering food from its natural state is problematic. However, by definition a food that is frozen, refrigerated, dehydrated or prepared with sanitary measures is *processed*. Pasteurized milk is processed to kill microorganism contaminants such as TB. It is true that refined white flour, instead of whole grains, is often added to pasta, and sodium is frequently used as a preservative and for flavor in canned goods. Obviously, Fruit Loops is not on the Paleo Diet.

Patients often ask me about diets, and I say it's less about what you eat and more about how much you consume. All diets work if they provide fewer calories than required by the patient's body, and result in weight loss and health benefits which justify the effort.

Every year the US News and World Report reviews and ranks the numerous diets available. Also, Healthline.com offers a useful guide of the various options. The highest rated diet for cardiovascular health is the TLC (Therapeutic Lifestyle Changes Diet) developed by the NIH to lower the bad (LDL) cholesterol by restricting saturated fats. Also, the DASH diet receives high marks by lowering salt consumption and improving blood pressure control.

Every year the Weight Watchers program and Jenny Craig diet plans score very high marks through portion control, education and motivation. Diets like the Glycemic Index, South Beach and NutriSystem focus on limiting sugar, and emphasize lean protein choices and lower caloric intake. Some believe that Americans can adopt the Mediterranean Diet of southern Italy, Greece and Crete and have the same improved outcomes. This diet emphasizing vegetables, fruit, olive oil, fish and poultry is sensible, especially if washed down with the advised red wine! However, the ancestry of southern Europe is different than the southern United States. Perhaps it's the moonshine instead of the wine.

Other diets include the high protein and low carbohydrate Atkins diet, the low fat and low carbohydrate Scarsdale diet, the low fat and vegetarian Dean Ornish, and many others including the goofy New Beverly Hills diet and the Grapefruit diet. My personal favorite for ridiculous is The Skinny Bitch Diet. The latter is essentially a vegan diet without dairy, caffeine, sugar or alcohol. I can see how this diet gets its name. The French have a philosophy that you are what you eat. For diets to work, it should be you are what you don't eat.

I remain fascinated by medicine and the wonders of The Creation. Basic science research arguably seems foolish at times, but sometimes it connects the dots. How did our hunter gatherer ancestors survive before the earth warmed, allowing farming and animal husbandry to provide us a more reliable food supply? In the Paleolithic era a kill of a large animal might provide food for a few days. A survival advantage would occur if those precious calories could be assimilated, stored and then carefully doled out during lean periods. The thrifty gene hypothesis holds that the insulin molecule evolved to give that survival edge.

A recent discovery adds to our knowledge of our ancestor's gluttony-starvation cycle. The intestinal Paneth cell has been described as "the most beautiful cell of the human body" because of its appearance under the microscopic lens. However, research suggests that the Paneth cell's beauty may also come from the explanation of why cycles of fasting in our modern age seem to promote greater weight gain as dieting ends. It appears that calorie restriction causes the Paneth cell to prime the intestinal cells for re-feeding. When this occurs in our land of plenty a burst of cellular growth results and the intestine is quickly transformed to greater absorptive efficiency.

As Spock would say, "Fascinating"!

Cramps - October 29, 2009

People tell me their stories and I've heard a lot of stories over forty years. I've learned to listen with the mind and the heart. In medical school I was taught physiology (how the body works) and how diseases change those normal functions. My professors emphasized the value of associating diseases with people and their stories. But I have to admit that I resisted those lessons. I tended to focus on the disease more than the person. It was only later as I developed relationships with my patients and experienced their suffering that I came to understand the wisdom of everyone's unique story.

Internists are mechanistic creatures. They want to know **why** something happens, and the why hopefully leads to **what** to do about the problem. Cases in point are the common conditions of *leg cramps*, *heart failure* and a *stiff neck*. You may be surprised to read that all of these conditions are related by a basic mechanism. Neck pain is common and I frequently explain to patients why their necks hurt and what they need to do about it. It was during a visit to my daughter in Portland that a better way of communicating the problem came to me as I was strolling along the Willamette River.

I suspect that many of you have seen teams of rowers in shells on the Tennessee River. These long narrow boats are propelled by teams of rowers who pull synchronously at long oars under the direction of the coxswain (the pilot). Now imagine a muscle composed of many muscle fibers like a rope made of many strands. Next imagine even smaller muscle units called fibrils that are in turn composed of parallel proteins comparable to the shells with their rowers. I'm able to move my fingers across the key board and type this essay because tiny strands of proteins called myosin bind to and pull against another tiny parallel protein called actin, much as rowers pull their oars against the water and move the shell forward. Neat, huh!

It turns out that muscles work best when there is teamwork and optimal positioning of the myosin and actin proteins. It's like having all the oars in the water and everyone pulling together to produce maximum power and efficiency. A basic mechanism of muscle dysfunction results when a non-optimal relationship of these parallel proteins develops. I vividly remember an experiment in medical school where we measured the force of contraction of a muscle. We then progressively stretched the muscle and measured an even stronger force of contraction as a result of a better alignment of the proteins. Why do you think athletes warm up and stretch prior to a game? It's to stretch their muscles and muscle fibers, and to optimally align the myosin and actin proteins at the cellular level.

Ultimately, there comes a point where further stretching passes the point of optimal alignment and the power of contraction decreases. A researcher named Frank Starling discovered the basic physiology of heart failure known as Starling's Law. A fundamental treatment for heart failure is the use of a diuretic that removes excess fluid from the body and decreases the heart's size. The decrease in heart size realigns the muscle fibers in a more efficient relationship. Night time cramps in calves are also common and are associated with tired and energy-depleted muscles as well as fluid and electrolyte (sodium and potassium) shifts. The treatment is stretching the cramping muscle along its long axis. Prevention measures include stretching at bedtime and avoiding fluid imbalance like edema.

The mechanism and treatment of sore neck muscles is virtually the same, but posture is emphasized as a preventive strategy. I tell patients to imagine a Harlem Globetrotter who spins a basketball on his fingertip. I tell patients to make sure their head is centered on the neck analogous to the basketball.

I once read that flexibility correlates with health. It seems that as I get older I find myself needing to stretch the muscles from my neck down and even down to my sore plantar fascia (soles of my feet). I certainly don't want to lose the flexibility in my neck that allows me to look backwards over my shoulder enabling me to safely back my truck out of the garage. And I certainly don't want my daughters to someday insist that I get one of those commercial beepers that sound when my truck is in reverse. That would really cramp me up!

One of my favorite authors is Isaac Asimov. I began reading him because he's a science fiction writer like me, only more successful! It was later that I discovered he was a polymath. This is a modern word for what was once called a "Renaissance Man," or a person who is schooled in many disciplines. Leonardo da Vinci was such a man. Asimov has published books on every topic in the Dewey decimal library system. In my own library I have Asimov books of science fiction, humor, basic science, interpretations of Shakespeare's plays, and a 1200-page commentary on the Bible.

When my children were young they would often come to me with questions. I quickly learned that the answers needed to be short ones without digressions or pontification. I would often tell them that the answer they sought might require several sentences and then ask them if they really wanted their question answered. Not infrequently they would roll their eyes and say, "That's OK, Dad."

The word doctor derives from the Latin word docere. It means to teach, and that's what I do. I teach my patients about their problems while answering their questions. I teach nurses, even colleagues and my children when possible. I look forward to teaching my grandson who will be born in May 2012. And I teach my readers of the Knoxville Focus. People ask me why I bother to write each week. I do so because it gives me joy and because I'm a teacher at heart.

I also enjoy public speaking which is another aspect of teaching. This form of instruction once terrified me. My nature is not a thespian like my wife. She is energized when on stage; it's hard work for me. Early in my career I found that my fear of public speaking was a hindrance so I practiced and practiced, even memorizing entire lectures before going to the podium. I can do it now with ease. A friend recently told me that my recent presentation to his Sunday school class was wonderful, and that I "had a gift." No, it is hard work that makes it look natural and easy, even without a teleprompter.

Have you ever seen yourself in a video or heard your recorded voice? We see and hear ourselves differently than others do. You often hear people say they don't like having their picture taken which means their vision of themselves is different from that of others or the camera. My daughter is in her last trimester and she looks pregnant. I told her that it's hard for a woman to comprehend how differently men and woman visualize pregnancy. Apparently, genetic imprinting in a man helps him to see a pregnant woman as attractive where women see only their... bigness.

A corollary to these musings is my objectivity concerning my own writing. I've found that I leave out words because I know what I'm trying to say and my eyes just imagine the words on the page. Fortunately, I have an editor, who reads over my work, corrects my omissions, and makes sure my modifiers aren't misplaced. My wife Becky has been modifying my behavior for the thirty-six years of our marriage, and now edits these *homemade* stories.

Last week I looked into the mirror and I looked… old. Perhaps it was because my dictation device had ruffled my hair, but it seemed more than just a bad hair day. Maybe it was the stress of the Obama-care mandated electronic medical records that add an extra hour and fifteen minutes to my ten and a half hour professional days. Maybe it was because I no longer have as much time to spend teaching patients about their medical problems and discussing their concerns, because I now have to retreat to my office and do "point and click" data entry on the EMR system. Maybe I'm just tired of fighting the Knoxville City government who continues to torment us as we try and improve our property. Maybe, like the Psalmist, I'm having trouble "singing the Lord's song in [an increasingly] foreign land."

As I listen to the purported *news* manipulated by the perverse media, and parse the rhetoric of the candidates and the pundits, I lament the class warfare brought to the homeland by our own President.

I've searched the world for a place to relocate and escape, but, like Socrates, I concluded that I cannot abandon my homeland. I may be forced to drink the hemlock, but one day freedom will again spring up from my ashes. By then I will be "free at last, free at last…"

Some days it's easier to write than others. Today it's tough because I have lots of things to do on this gorgeous spring afternoon. Murphy's Law states that the job at hand expands to fill the time allotted. My corollary to this law is that a job not only fills, but overruns the time available. As I look back, I don't know how I got anything else done while I was managing a large medical practice!

I love the "new" green colors of spring which emerge after the dormancy of winter. I've begun to see butterflies, and last week I was surprised to see lightening bugs on "tax day." I don't think these early signs of spring have anything to do with global warming or the hyping of the recent "blood moon." Today I found ants on my peonies. We sometimes think of ants as pests, but they are necessary and these beautiful southern flowers won't open without ants doing their work. Did you know there are three pronunciations of peonies? There is the sophisticated French like *pee-oh-knees*. Then there is the southern *pee-OH-knees* as my grandmother used to say. And lastly we have the countrified *pie-knees*.

My garden is already plowed and planting has begun there and in the pastures of our small farm. Even the horses have a spring in their step with the changing weather and perhaps as their diet shifts from hay to the tender new grass. My grandson, Oakley may also have "spring fever" because he constantly tells us he wants to "go outside." There's a lot to entertain a little boy "outside" on a farm.

Some years ago I wrote an essay describing winter as especially tough on the frail. This is certainly true in nature because there is no medical care for injured animals. However, winter is also tough for humans despite our support systems. We live in a dangerous world, but due to the wondrous design of our bodies we are able to grub in the dirt of a garden, muck horse stalls, and rarely suffer serious harm even as we endure the pollen of spring. This is possible as long as the defense systems of our skin and our immune system function properly. These systems do age along with the rest of the body, and even young and robust souls can be overwhelmed.

I've been thinking about viruses lately with the resurgence of the dreaded Ebola virus epidemic in West Africa. Viruses are very primitive entities that we don't even classify as life forms, principally because they cannot reproduce without a plant or animal host. These invaders cause harm when our defenses are overcome and our cell walls are breached. The Trojan Horse was similarly a *lifeless* structure, but was deadly to ancient Trojans because it was filled with lurking Greek warriors who emerged to wreak havoc.

Apparently, computers are subject to "viruses" of a different type, referred to by my computer guy as malware. In medicine "mal" refers a diseased condition or sickness, as in malformation or malnourishment. There is also malpractice that connotes injury to a patient when a doctor violates the standards of medical care. Recently my computer's defenses were overwhelmed. Computer-Doc's diagnosis was infestation by no less than six "Trojan viruses" – and the treatment to eliminate this infestation has been rough on us all.

I'm not alone in this post-modern world of high tech and "Trojan malware." According to security experts, even the Obama-care website is vulnerable to *viruses* like the "Heartbleed" malware currently making the rounds. Last week a friend of mine reported that her computer suddenly flashed a message from Homeland Security which said her computer had been flagged for surfing pornography! She was told to go to Wal-Mart and purchase software to fix the problem. My friend is too sharp to fall for this ruse and far too fine a lady to have been "surfing porn," so instead she took her machine to the computer ER. After a $300 resuscitation, a cure was pronounced and the *patient* was discharged home. Unfortunately, the treatment was incomplete because on her next visit to the internet, my virtuous friend was contacted by Interpol, the International Criminal Police Organization, again with the charge of driving her computer in a "bad neighborhood!"

I've learned through all these misadventures to appreciate the security guardians who protect us. I've also come to understand that to survive in the 21st century you not only need a good doctor and a reliable car mechanic, but also an available plumber and a first rate computer geek. I've also learned to regularly check my computer's security program which I envision as analogous to a sentry in the army or a watchman on the wall made famous in modern times by the soliloquy of Jack Nicholson's character in the movie **A Few Good Men**.

In ancient times people often lived near walled cities for protection and a watchman's duty was to stand guard on those walls and look for approaching danger. When the exiled Hebrews returned to Jerusalem, Nehemiah led his people to rebuild the protecting wall around the city. Tradition holds that he worked with a trowel in one hand and a spear in the other as he kept watch for enemies.

Some years ago a friend of mine awarded me the honorific title of "watchman." There are many references to watchmen in the Bible ranging from ordinary men to prophets. I certainly don't count myself with the latter group. Some might just aver that I've got a big mouth. Actually, I don't have a bully pulpit like the President. All I have is the Focus to continue to sound the alarm as I have done for the last five years. However, what good is a watchman if no one listens or heeds his warnings?

It has been twenty years since I was in this place which is like no other. The last time I was in Yellowstone it was as a side trip with my children. The girls had wanted to go to a dude ranch. I found a dude ranch on the northern boundary of Yellowstone, and so we compromised. We did the dude ranch, and I took them to a place of wonder. Now, it was our thirty-sixth wedding anniversary, and this time Becky and I skipped the dude ranch and instead did the Grand Tetons and Yellowstone.

These two national parks are less than fifty miles apart and must be on everyone's bucket list. It's relatively easy to get to Jackson Hole, Wyoming, which is surrounded by the postcard Grand Tetons; and Yellowstone is only an hour up the road. I have a saying: "Get on a plane, rent a car, and you can see the world."

Becky and I have adventurous spirits, and we like to stay on the go. I've told her that we can do and see more in four days than the average twosome can in a week. I could tell you about beautiful Jenny Lake, with my daughter's namesake, and the best hikes I've ever taken. I could tell you about surprising a moose with a huge rack lounging under a tree not thirty feet from the trail. I could tell you about buffalo all around our car, elk grazing on meadows surrounded by steaming fumaroles, or a black bear scampering along a ridge line. But, what I really wanted to tell you about is the *healing* of the Earth.

In 1988 one third of Yellowstone burned despite a massive firefighting effort. Lightning strikes had ignited forest fires which were fueled by underbrush that had been allowed to accumulate rather than being periodically burnt away by Mother Nature. Man's well intentioned policy of fire suppression sought to protect our forests, but Smokey the Bear did not understand the consequences. It took a late summer squall and a half inch of snow to put out the fires that man and his technology had been unable to squelch for months. I remember the cries of outrage directed at the fire policy of the National Forest Service and the comments of the media which said that Yellowstone was gone forever. And they were wrong, again.

When my family was there twenty years ago the experts were just starting to have second thoughts about the forest fires, as the recovery had already begun in Yellowstone. Beautiful fireweed, similar to Indian paintbrush, was springing up from the charred forest floor, and lodgepole pine began sprouting from seeds released from cones opened by fire. Just as the resin on the cones of the mighty Sequoyah is melted by fire, releasing packets of precious genetic material for the next generation, Yellowstone's pine forests are similarly designed with fire in mind.

They better be because they live on a volcano. Six hundred and thirty-four thousand years ago a volcano erupted in Yellowstone that was estimated to be 1000 times as large as the eruption of Mount St. Helens. As the cataclysmic eruption progressed, the center of the volcano collapsed upon itself and produced a depression in its center called a caldera. This 30 by 40 mile depression became the Yellowstone basin and ultimately our national park. Scientists tell us that the Yellowstone volcano is still active, having also erupted 2.5 million and 1.2 million years ago, and will erupt again. When it does the Park will cease to exist as we know it, but like the forest, it will rise again like a Phoenix.

I've always been a conservationist, even before it was cool. Several years ago I happened to run into a liberal friend of mine twice in one month at a recycling center. Both times he expressed amazement that a conservative would recycle. What foolish bias, I thought. The very word conservative comes from the root Latin word meaning to conserve traditions and the natural way of things.

Mankind's big problem is hubris, what the ancient Greeks called arrogant pride. In fact, the greatest sin in ancient Greek culture was hubris. We moderns think we're smart, and we are the smartest creatures who have ever existed on this planet. But, the Universe is vast, and the Earth is a huge and very complex biosphere. We should be good stewards, but our reliance on technology, our finite knowledge, and our institutions will only go so far and our pride keeps getting us into trouble as has happened before throughout history.

I'm sorry if this week's offering is a bit preachy or sounds like a travelogue, but I write about what's on my heart. So, I'll leave you with a *green* perspective that isn't artificial, politically correct, or impractical like switchgrass fuels. The picture below is God's healing forest. This green works every time.

Sometimes I have trouble remembering whether I've told a story or just thought about it. Stories are so much a part of me that they bubble up when prompted. I don't want to be repetitious, but I also don't like to peruse my old essays because I'm rarely satisfied with the words I've chosen, the syntax or even the sentences I've constructed. A friend once asked me about a quotation I used as a chapter header in my novel *Epiphany.* I looked it up and found that I used the quotation correctly. Unfortunately, my eyes drifted downward over my novel's prose and I found that I didn't like much of what I'd written. Perhaps that's a bit strong, but I've discovered that I have to accept my essays when the newspaper's deadline arrives, and accept that the work was the best I could do at that moment.

As cold season is upon us I wanted to challenge you with the story of how *far fomites can fly.* "What the heck's a fomite?" you might ask. Hang on and you'll find out.

I'm sure all of you have observed how sunlight can sometimes reflect and illuminate dust particles floating in the air. I find it magical when we see things in a different light and in a different way. I once observed two friends in a conversation in front of a window with the early morning sunlight streaming in around them. They were speaking calmly, and yet I could clearly see tiny droplets of spittle (fomites) coming from their mouths as they spoke, and cascading downward showcased in the light. I've seen similar eruptions from singers.

The scientist in me yearned to measure the exact horizontal distance those droplets traveled, but this would have been…peculiar in a social setting. Suffice it to say, I would estimate that a person could avoid conversational spray if they stayed at arm's reach. An old Seinfeld show spoofed people who stand much too close. Beware of *close-talkers* in the flu season! The safe zone might even be smaller if you were seated and someone was standing over you and lecturing or singing. In that case, the droplets might travel a greater distance – like rocks thrown over a cliff – before hitting your face. Yuck!

I'm sure all of you can see the practical aspects of these observations especially during the cold and flu season. We all know it's best to wash our hands, use hand sanitizers, and cough or sneeze into our sleeves rather than into our hands or a handkerchief. Fortunately, few people these days carry a handkerchief like my dad used to carry in his hip pocket. Viruses are spread by uncovered coughs and by contact with infected surfaces like someone's handshake. I'll bet you have a new appreciation of your personal space after hearing this story! There's no need to be paranoid, just common-sensical. Just be aware of the world around you, including others who might not be so careful with their sneezes and coughs.

To what extent are we aware of the world around us? Do we see superficially or do we see with the trained eyes of experience? Wisdom writings say that we "see dimly as if in a mirror," and as a result we overlook important aspects of a situation or make snap judgments about what we perceive as right. An example is throwing money at poverty or blaming others for the consequences of our poor choices.

Perhaps my bad cold and month of misery was a blessing in disguise that I can now comprehend. The ancient Greeks thought that the greatest sin was hubris – arrogant pride. I don't fancy myself as arrogant or *excessively* prideful, but perhaps being humbled occasionally is good for the soul. To stand on the edge of the abyss changes one's perspective and has refocused me on what is most important in life.

I still get up every morning, do my devotional, and go to work; but now I'm a bit more reverent of every day I'm given.

I've often mentioned that my escape reading is science fiction. In the famous science fiction novel *Dune* by Frank Herbert there comes a critical moment where the protagonist looks upward and passionately shouts, "Father, the sleeper has awakened." Yes, how true.

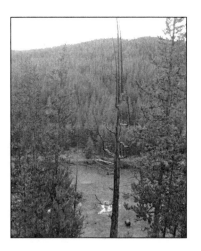

For a long time I've had a metaphoric vision of my life as a cross-country airplane trip. As a young man I packed my bags and hustled to the airport to make my life-flight. I fastened my seat belt by buckling down in college before racing down the runway and soaring into the sky of medical school. Pretty soon I reached cruising altitude of marriage, family, and medical practice. There have been bumps and turbulence along the way, but Becky and I have been blessed.

When flying you can sense when the pilot begins his descent. I've now reached that point and have begun a slow, controlled descent toward my ultimate destination. I can now envision a final approach to my destination *airport* where I will land and then taxi to the hanger for old planes. Fortunately, that's still a ways off because I now envision leaving the dysfunctional medical system and beginning a concierge medical practice where my patients and I will again be in control of their medical care.

Years ago I read a fascinating book by William Strauss and Neil Howe called, **Generations, The History of America's Future, 1584 to 2069.** The title itself intrigued me as I wondered how a book tracing the history of America could predict its future. The authors discovered that each generation has a mood and characteristics. An example is the *Greatest Generation* who came of age during the Second World War and won it. Interestingly, this cohort of Americans has many of the characteristics of the Founders of our country who fought and won America's freedom. As a *Baby Boomer* it's interesting to consider the characteristics we have in common with the generation of The Great Awakening (c.1740) and the Transcendental Movement (c.1830).

Recently, a young co-worker of the *Millennial Generation* pleasantly advised me not to fret about my patients demanding unnecessary tests. She said it was time for Baby Boomers like me to transfer control and decision making to the next generation. She said her cohort would not have a problem saying, "No" to seniors with unreasonable expectations. Coincidentally, another Millennial told me he couldn't afford to be pessimistic about Obama and the country because he had fifty years in his future. Their perspectives challenged me as I reminisced over my earlier life as a rising professional and family man. At that time I thought I was in charge of some things. Perhaps we're all adjusting to the new order and its realities.

Strauss and Howe defined a generation as twenty-two years and showed how generational types have repeated themselves throughout American history. In fact, the generational types have marched in order since our ancestors came to North America in the sixteen hundreds. Even more intriguing is the author's finding that America has been alternately challenged by external threats (WW II) or internal conflicts (the turbulent sixties) about every forty-four years. And if history does repeat itself, America is due to experience another external challenge that will begin in 2014.

As I observe America tear itself apart with perpetual race conflicts, foreign wars, ruinous Washington spending, IRS and other government scandals, and liberal versus conservative politics, all manipulated by a media that has long hence sold its soul, I wonder if we're going to enter another Civil War. The one thing that gives me hope is that America has risen to challenges over the last 400 years, and the *Millennial Generation* has much in common with the *Greatest Generation* who created the United States and saved the world from Nazi Germany.

Western Civilization was a required course in my college cohort. The course terrorized many, but I found it fascinating to consider why western culture succeeded. A recent book by Rodney Stark, **The Triumph of Reason,** maintains that Western Civilization is the product of Christian philosophy. This perspective holds that every individual is unique and loved by God. This empowering notion allowed western man to create and prosper like no civilization in history.

In Western culture the individual is more than an ant who serves its colony. Because western man recognized an Absolute (God), he possessed a standard by which to measure what is right, what is moral or virtuous. Our post-modern era holds that there are no absolutes and everything is relative. When the Absolute is replaced by the "arbitrary absolutes" of man, then anything goes and is ruled by the majority sentiment of the moment. And as truth/facts are manipulated by the "arbitrary elites" of the media, is it any wonder that we're in trouble? Incidentally, another philosophy of our post-modernism is the triumph of "style over substance," apparently aided by teleprompters.

C.S. Lewis spoke of the devolution of Western culture in his 1944 book the **Abolition of Man.** Later, George Orwell's **1984** showed the dystopian result of the renunciation of absolutes. Ayn Rand's **Atlas Shrugged** echoed Orwell. And Francis Schaeffer in **How Should We Then Live** explained the end result of liberal progressive humanist philosophy that now indoctrinates our children in schools, and permeates entertainment and our government. Those who read history and think independently know what is wrong and major surgery is needed.

Perhaps the next generation is the way out of our mess. Admittedly, we *Baby Boomers* have focused excessively on ourselves and often neglected our civic duty. The pursuit of "personal peace and affluence" led to Rome rotting from the inside.

Ayn Rand once told a story of a magnificent tree which suddenly fell to the ground during a storm. It was then discovered that the tree was rotten at its center. I only hope this isn't a metaphor for our country.

Lately, I've been thinking about entropy. Those readers who have taken courses in physics know that entropy is a fundamental principle of the universe. In fact, the second law of thermodynamics deals with entropy, and is the reason that time moves forward rather than in reverse.

Entropy is the process where all systems lose energy. An example is a spinning top that runs down or a battery that loses its charge over time. You might ask what this arcane principle of physics has to do with a column focused on medical issues. Well, if you accept the science behind entropy then read on and find out how this fundamental principle affects everything, including you.

Have you ever gone on vacation and discovered that when you return it takes a while to get back in the swing of things? I've noticed that when I return to my medical practice I sometimes have trouble remembering common drug dosages for a day or so. As a result I have to look up some dosages until I'm back up to speed. I've been in medicine for more than thirty-five years and yet the correct dosage of amoxicillin with clavulinic acid (*Augmentin*) fades after a week at the beach. You see my memory is subject to entropy.

This morning I exhorted (I strongly encouraged) my hospitalized patient to get out of bed. I know she felt bad, but I told her that her chest muscles don't work well when she stays in bed and this prolongs her recovery from pneumonia. I didn't mention entropy to her, but I told her that her muscles will become weaker if she stays in bed and doesn't use them vigorously. Perhaps I should have asked her to imagine treading water in the lake. If she quits treading she'll sink and drown.

Your body conserves energy, and this is germane to the first law of thermodynamics – we won't go into that today. The point is, use it or lose it! As an energy-conserving measure, muscle tissue is reabsorbed if it's not being used. As an example, if you put your arm in a sling the muscles will weaken and wither over time. If you send astronauts into space where there is no gravity, their muscles wither and their bones become osteoporotic. In fact, these problems are major obstacles to long space flights such as to another planet. Jesus called Lazarus out; I told Mrs. Jones – lovingly – to get the lead out!

The struggle to live is actually a struggle against entropy. We have to constantly forage and put food in our stomachs where the fats, proteins and carbohydrates are digested, absorbed and ultimately transported to the cells of our body to be *burned*. The released energy is used to drive our muscles and power our brains to think. Actually, all energy comes from the sun; we just harvest it.

The sun fuses hydrogen and releases vast amounts of energy which stream across space to warm the earth, drive photosynthesis in plants and begin the energy transfer process to us. Vegetarian animals feed on plants and we feed on plants and animals (we're omnivores). We actually feed on the sun's energy transferred to us through plants and animals. You'll be pleased to know that you also adhere to the first law of thermodynamics because none of us creates or destroys energy.

The 17th century philosopher, Rene Descartes, once said, "Cogito ergo sum" (I think therefore I am). He may be right, at least in part. The ancients held that existence came about when we were given the *breath of life*. Later, life was associated with a beating heart. We moderns think that being alive is associated with a functioning mind and our ability to think.

Spiritualists hold that the essence of a being resides within the soul. Did you know that those who die in a plane crash are referred to as "lost souls?" As a theist I can conceive of a *centered* place in my being that anatomically is unknown. The philosopher Emanuel Kant might have called this *numinous* (his term) spot the soul. The scientist/theist Blaise Pascal said, "There is a God-shaped vacuum in the heart of every person." And Mark Nebo envisions "an umbilical spot of Grace," which I picture as the place where my soul is tethered to the Creative and Sustaining Force of the universe.

What if the essence of a human is subject to entropy like everything else? The Master told us that we need *daily bread*, and I believe He meant not only victuals, but spiritual food.

I'm blessed to rarely hunger for food. However, I must work every day to feed my soul. Sadly, too many don't understand spiritual entropy and look for sustenance in drugs, money, power, politics and prestige.

Wisdom shows us that these baubles and idols never satisfy the deepest hunger or counter the effects of entropy.

Good Hair Day - October 31, 2009

"Doctor Ferguson, you look **hot** today!" I tried not to let my jaw drop or look foolish; after all, this young nurse was my friend and I could tell she was paying me a sincere compliment. In times past I might have said something to self-consciously dismiss her compliment and unintentionally insult the bearer of a gift. But, I've learned to accept these rare compliments because I've learned they are as good for the giver as the receiver.

Have you ever thought about how language changes? Words are the tools with which we express our thoughts. We use these tools to paint word pictures and to tell stories. Jesus was a master story teller who spoke in ancient Aramaic which was eventually translated into many other languages. You've heard it said that "Words matter" and this brings me back to my initial shock of being told that I'm *hot*. I have to admit that I was a bit shocked when I first heard someone described as *hot*. However, in the lexicon of 21st century America, this is a positive description and little more. Think about how we used the word *mouse* twenty-five years ago as compared to the present. Our language evolves; and so do we.

What was different about me that day which made my young friend take notice of a fifty-eight year old man? She said it was my hair and this caused me to think about what makes a "good hair day." Every day we get up, take a shower, comb our hair, and some days everything falls magically into place. On other days, despite our best efforts, our hair looks as though we stuck our finger into a light switch. My dermatology consultant on this issue tells me that our hair is constructed with disulfide bonds that curl when exposed to humidity. Well OK, but I sleep in an air-conditioned house with controlled humidity. Heat can also affect our hair, and so does static electricity; the latter is especially noticeable in drier, colder winter months. "Well, maybe you just slept on it in the right way," opined my consultant. I didn't tell him that I couldn't take a shower that fateful morning because the pump on our well blew out and I came to work with extra deodorant and my elbows tight to my sides.

It's hard for me to think of myself as *hot*. I try to take care of myself, though I've never looked into my mirror and asked "who's the fairest of them all?" I was once fat and vowed never to be fat again, so I walk regularly, take the stairs instead of the elevator, and consider whether every morsel is calorie-worthy.

I met my wife, Becky, in junior high school forty-three years ago. I worshipped her from afar because she moved in that rarefied air of grace that some girls just have. She said we were *friends* – that cursed moniker every male despises. We did date for a while as seniors in high school, but it was many years and experiences later that we found each other again and began our lives together – thirty-four years ago this September.

108

I don't pretend to understand why my *stock* went up in those intervening years. I'm just glad it did. I needed a life partner, an example of grace, and I believe it was arranged. You could say it was serendipity, but I hold it was more. I had more hair then; actually it was longer than hers in the early70's; but that was an era of "Long beautiful hair…shoulder length and longer."

Do you think that men are more *attractive* than women as they age? It certainly isn't true in all cases, but I hear this often enough to think many people hold this perspective. It certainly doesn't seem fair, but maybe the ledger sheet is finally being balanced by nature. From an evolutionary standpoint, younger women are more sought after when they are in their reproductive years, whereas older men are lauded for their maturity, even when they have less hair or bad hair.

Guys, the real trick is not to let things go to your head. Don't become an old fool as seems so commonplace these days – even if you're having a good hair day.

There's a saying among the French that you are what you eat. I remembered this perspective as I read an essay on gluten-sensitivity in the *Annals of Internal Medicine*. Researchers now believe that the spectrum of illness caused by sensitivity to the gluten component of wheat protein is much broader than I was taught thirty-five years ago. Doctors then understood celiac disease or gluten-sensitive enteropathy (intestinal disease) differently than today. This condition was defined more than a hundred years ago, but it took a Dutch physician in WW II to recognize that bread and cereals cause diarrhea in some people. And removing wheat products from the diet improved their diarrhea.

I find it fascinating that a similar chronic intestinal disorder was described in Turkey in the second century AD. The question is: has the world changed or did we? The world was much different twelve thousand years ago than it is today. Before the end of the last ice age people walked across the frozen Bering Land Bridge from Siberia and began to populate North America. Have you ever wondered why "native" Americans look so similar to those from the steps of Asia? We all came from somewhere and our first ancestors walked out of the Olduvai Gorge millions of years ago to populate the world, adapting as the climate demanded.

The final blasts of the ice age ended about 9600 BC. Hunter-gatherers no longer had to depend on the hunt because grains began to flourish in the Fertile Crescent as the earth warmed. Scientists have determined that a family gathering wild grain eight hours a day for three weeks could store enough grain for a year. No longer would our ancestors be forced to follow the wild herds; they could remain in one place and even plant their own grain and domesticate animals. One theory holds that religious perspectives arose out of those early collections of humans. Another theory holds that reverence for nature brought together divergent groups that would become the earliest civilizations.

Dietary wheat sensitivity has probably been around for a long time. However, we now have more sensitive diagnostic tests and are able to find problems before more serious disease occurs. The newest perspective is wheat sensitivity **without** objective tests or bowel disease. This is called nonceliac gluten-sensitivity. The symptoms are diarrhea, abdominal pain, bloating and excessive gas, headache, lethargy, mouth ulcers and even clumsiness or attention-deficit/hyperactivity disorder that improve with gluten withdrawal. A whole cottage industry has sprung up to help patients modify their diets, sell books, or malign modern wheat cultivation and wheat products.

I believe gluten-sensitive patients are accurately reporting their symptoms. There is a rare phenomenon called Munchausen's syndrome where people make up symptoms in order to have tests and surgery. This is a serious psychiatric problem and has no relationship to gluten-sensitivity syndrome. It is frustrating that our diagnostic precision is not perfect in gluten-sensitivity syndrome and perhaps it never will be. New perspectives and diagnostic clues for this enigmatic problem will arise as time goes on; in the meantime we do the best we can.

Much is also said these days about hunger in America. I wonder how Americans can be hungry despite the fact that two-thirds of us are overweight or obese. Michelle Obama has been on a mission to educate our people about healthy eating habits. Perhaps the tendency to obesity is in our genes.

Imagine a clan of hunter-gatherers tens of thousands of years ago who have just brought down a wooly mammoth. Conceivably, there's a survival advantage to being able to consume large quantities of food and store those calories for lean times, and then to parsimoniously release the stored reserves to power bodily functions. The adaptive hormone of this *thrifty gene hypothesis* (the storage of food energy during times of plenty) is insulin. Perhaps our modern problem is that we live in a land of plenty, but have the genes of hunter-gatherers.

So what do we do? We don't have the science or the wisdom to alter our DNA. However, we are rational beings and if you eat something and it makes you sick, stop eating it, even though avoiding gluten is expensive and difficult. And if you realize that your body is designed to prevent starvation, don't overfeed it. It's not rocket science and the government shouldn't take away our liberty to order a large soft drink.

I suspect that President Obama gets tired of Michelle's arugula because I've heard he sometimes slips off for a hot dog with chili. My recommendation is be sensible. Don't gorge on hot dogs every day, or wash down your super-sized fries with a large regular Coke! The Bible teaches moderation in everything.

Food for thought...and consumption.

Even after fifty years I can still see the red dirt outlined by the carefully manicured grass and the bluest sky I've ever seen. It was a magical day as my Mom and Dad led me down the aisle to our seats at Crosley Field in Cincinnati. It was 1959 and I was eight years old and it was my first Big League Baseball game. I tasted my first ball park hot dog that day, and it wasn't pink. And I discovered that mustard was not always a French's yellow. I've watched major league baseball in five other ball parks since then, including The House that Ruth Built, but nothing compares to that first ball park memory.

Is there anything more American than baseball or the 4th of July? Whether you like baseball or not, it is a slice of Americana. You may argue that baseball is played in other places, but the game started here and it is our National pastime. Now, calm down, I also love other sports including football and golf, but on this 4th of July I'm focusing on things uniquely American such as Friday night high school football, apple pie, and marching bands at halftime, even though I don't particularly care for them.

Perhaps, it's the relatively slow pace of baseball that I like. As Becky and I watch the Braves or the Smokies, there's time for conversation and even time to go to the refreshment stand or use the facilities without resorting to the TiVo pause button on the remote.

We all live at such a frenzied pace. I love the old Andy Griffith show that depicts an idealized America with front porches, family values and Sunday lunches after church. I'm sure other cultures have nostalgic customs like picnics or even summertime vacations at the beach with family and friends. But I'm not a relativist; I believe in America. I also believe in the ideal which produces the notions of morality and virtue. In fact, these visions of reality are foundational for me and give meaning to my life.

America is not perfect; no human institution is. Our Western culture, though based on Judeo-Christian precepts, has made mistakes. But, when we Americans make mistakes we are remorseful for the miscarriages of authority or the violation of the ideals of our Founding Fathers.

I've always been interested in the notion of conscience. Do you remember the little cartoon angel that sits on one shoulder urging you to ignore the little devilish muse that whispers into the opposite ear? Conscience makes you consider others beyond yourself and what is the right thing to do. I suspect conscience is a universal aspect of all humans, but I can only speak for myself and my Country. I can tell you that something inside me urges me to listen to God's spirit. And I answer to that Voice, to myself, and to my wife, in that order. The very fact that I measure myself against the Ideal, rather than the man-made contrivances of State or Party, keeps me from rationalizing my behavior or merely comparing myself to those around me. Now, don't get me wrong, I screw up like everyone else, so I dutifully account for my efforts at the end of each day to my Maker. I relish the fact that I still live in a free country with choices and consequences. And I get my marching orders every morning from the Ideal, not from Washington.

So, on this day that celebrates our Country and our freedoms, bought at such a terrible cost, I will bow my head and say thanks as I celebrate with hot dogs and my family. And it is thankfulness that encourages me to serve. And you know what? I'm not ashamed of my country, our culture, and the good that we've done in the world. In fact, I'm sick and tired of our politicians apologizing and denigrating the United States.

Therefore, on this 4th of July I resolve not to feel guilty, but to be thankful and answer the call to serve others. I resolve to "speak the truth in love" and ignore the perverse media. And I will declare that I don't care what the Mullahs think about us.

My wife, Becky, relates a story of a long departed relative who grew up in the Great Depression. This lady understood privation, and as a result saved everything for the proverbial "rainy day." As the family sorted through her life's history and estate (collections) they found a box full of tiny pieces of string. The box was labeled, "strings too short to tie."

Becky is a good steward of God's blessings. We waste very little, not because we know poverty, but because we feel it's the right thing to do. Some years ago I ran into a self-described modern-liberal-progressive friend at a recycling center. He looked at me with a puzzled expression and then asked what I was doing there. Perhaps it was Paul's description of patience (one "fruit of the Spirit" (Galatians 5:22) that caused me to merely reply, "Conservatives recycle too." In fact, I was recycling long before it was cool.

Becky is the manager of our home and she maintains that my semi-retirement has not infringed on her space. Her center of operations is her kitchen, and though I visit to help, I would never deign to rearrange – I love rhyming words for emphasis. Recently, my daughter obtained permission to rearrange some drawers in our home that she found teeming with clutter. She found no boxes of "string too short to tie," but almost. And the good news, The Mistress of the House was pleased with the organizational results.

Recently, a crisis occurred on our small Thistle Farm. Our latest project is remodeling an out-building and converting it to a hen house for eggs. Becky loves eggs; I don't. Long ago on a trip to Europe before medical school, I found myself far from home, sick, and convalescing in a cheap *pension* in Madrid. The standard fare at the hostelry was gazpacho and egg dishes. At one time or another, most of us have associated an illness with a certain food. I survived my "Spanish flu," and can now tolerate gazpacho, but egg dishes bring back unwelcome memories. It is my opinion that eggs should be reserved for pastry or Hollandaise sauce.

But I digress. Our crisis was a raccoon who was killing our chickens. I have a tender heart and as a result I no longer hunt. I realize this may be a bit hypocritical because I now forage at Kroger. However, as penance I say a prayer for the animal that gave its life for me.

Raccoons are very resourceful creatures and our "coon" was not to be deterred by an otherwise secure chicken house. Farm living is educational, and as we searched for a raccoon solution we discovered that even the Have-a-Heart trap we purchased to capture and relocate the intruder was not enough. The authorities we contacted informed us that trapped raccoons should be "exterminated" because they can transmit rabies. Alternatively, we could try to transport the coon if we were successful trapping it, but taking our problem to another person's property seemed problematic.

I've written about our dog Jack in other Focus essays. He's a mountain feist and bred to hunt squirrels. I discovered this breeding apparently extends to raccoons as well when a ruckus erupted in our front yard. Jack had treed the murderous raccoon and a conundrum ensued. Reluctantly, the ex-hunter was brought out of retirement and became the temporary coon hunter to end the chicken killing spree. And that's where the kitchen drawer enters the story.

Good writing holds the reader in suspense, so hang on, Folks. Some have asked me where my stories come from. The famous comedian Will Rogers was asked the same. He replied, "I don't make jokes. I just watch the government and report the facts!"

My problem with hunting is less about ethics than the fact that you often don't dispatch your prey instantly with one shot. And so it was with the coon who was knocked out of the tree by my shot gun blast only to be attacked by my mutt. All I could hear as I made my way through the dense brush were frenzied yelps and ferocious snarls. I found the two adversaries locked in mortal combat, a veritable blur of roiling, instinctual hatred. I managed to separate the two long enough to send one to its Maker and the other to the makeshift trauma center in the middle of Becky's kitchen.

With any trauma, the ER staff quickly assesses the patient's condition and injuries. Jack was bloodied, but not seriously hurt. He had, however, sacrificed a frontal incisor (tooth) to the battle. We sometimes refer to Jack as "Uncle Jack" because his father is his brother. Breeders often violate human laws of consanguinity to propagate favorable traits such as treeing squirrels and barking like a fool so the hunter can harvest the game. Unfortunately, selective breeding also produced Jack's prominent under-bite. Now, he sports a hillbilly dental array as well.

As we worked on our wounded family member in our make-shift ER, I searched for equipment necessary for his evaluation and treatment. Where else should I look, but The Kitchen Drawer?

The saga ended with a prayer for the departed coon and laughter. Our family "LOL" (laughed out loud) at Jack's new look. I won't show you the other picture Becky and I sent to the family of us wearing the fake teeth I found in Becky's kitchen drawer while searching for bandages.

The moral of this story? Never underestimate the resources of a kitchen drawer and save the fake teeth you find in there. You never know when you'll need them.

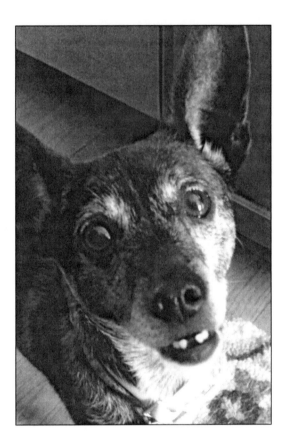

Consanguinity (and the rest of Jack's story)

"What kind of dog is that?" asked Ms. S as I greeted her at my front door. She was seeing me for concierge medical care and was obviously puzzled by my dog Jack. I explained to her that Jack is a Mountain Feist, but he is actually a "rescue."

In my previous life and practice I had a patient who bred feists as squirrel hunting dogs. My nurse of many years holds a tender spot for all creatures, and agrees with George Orwell's pigs in **Animal Farm** who maintained, "Four legs good, two legs...[not so good]." As LuAnn checked the breeder's blood pressure she learned of a runt in the new litter of pups, and it "wasn't going to make it." LuAnn was horrified to discover that breeder's often cull undesirables. The runt needed another option, and so he became our Jack.

Jack's genes are evident when a squirrel enters our yard because he goes ballistic and promptly trees the bushy-tailed rodent who dared challenge his range. Jack is also quick to greet anyone who comes to our farm, though he loses interest quickly unless you have a bushy tail. I've told Becky that our adopted "child" would make a wonderful greeter at Wal-Mart.

As I was relating Jack's story, Mrs. S was patting his head, but then inquired about Jack's pronounced under-bite. And that's where this week's essay began. I told her that Jack also goes by the name, "Uncle Jack" because his father is also his brother! I've learned that breeders frequently violate the laws of **consanguinity**. This is a term describing blood relatives or descendants. In the Middle Ages it was recognized that children of close relatives can produce genius, but more often idiocy. The prohibition of marrying closer than a fourth cousin derives from these observations, and subsequently became part of English Common Law. I haven't discussed the taboos of consanguinity with Jack.

Humans are inquisitive creatures. In fact, this inquisitive nature may have induced us to explore our environment and perhaps stimulated the development of reason. There is something about us that makes us want to know "Why?" My wife Becky loves mystery stories; I do not, but I am intrigued by the "why" of things. However, I've observed an inherent danger in explanations. People and doctors sometimes blindly accept explanations and stop inquiring and thinking.

The recent murderous rampage in Santa Barbara, California again raises the question "Why?" Mental illness is a quick answer, but I believe it's far more complicated. As a parent I empathized with the murderer's parents who apparently tried to help their dysfunctional son who was said to have "high functioning Asperger's Syndrome." Was mental illness the cause or just our collective need to explain why he chose to kill others and then himself?

A scientific paper on autism spectrum disorders (ADS) in the May 2014 JAMA (Journal of the American Medical Association) seems timely. These disorders are defined by impaired social interaction and communication as well as restricted interests and repetitive behaviors (Hollander, Textbook of Autism Spectrum Disorders). Apparently, ASD affects 1-2% of children in the general population, and includes Asperger's Syndrome, considered by the American Psychiatric Association to be a mild form of ASD. I read some years ago that there was speculation that Bill Gates has "high functioning" Asperger's Syndrome.

What is normal behavior? This is not a rhetorical question. How long does it take you to realize something or someone is not right? If you trust your instincts I'll bet it doesn't take long to conclude someone is dysfunctional. When I was a boy we had a beautiful white Persian cat who my mother euphemistically named Marilyn after Marilyn Monroe. Neither of these Marilyns was "right." The beautiful cat would sit in a mud puddle and birds would flock to our yard to swoop at poor Marilyn until she escaped their torment by huddling under a bush. And the cat's namesake was so impaired that she killed herself.

Discernment is a part of human nature, but what if we override our common sense? We accept a wide variation of "normal," and that's good. I've often quipped, "It's good to be a mongrel." How tragic it would be if we were all bred to tree squirrels or judged by Aryan standards. Our problem is that political correctness and the attempt to mandate equality has run amok. It now trumps common sense, and has begun to endanger us all. What if political correctness prevents us from saying someone is dangerous to himself or others? We once had institutions where impaired people were sheltered and treated. Now these folks are out on the street talking to themselves, selling their bodies for drugs and sometimes preying upon each other. Our political correctness causes us to strip-search granny at the airport instead of profiling. And we set terrorists free. It's not the guns or knives that are dangerous. Pogo said it best, "We have met the enemy, and he is us."

Science can help us find our way if we don't close our minds to reason tempered by compassion and pragmatism. We can't legislate morality, but we can muster the courage to speak the truth in love and act accordingly.

The JAMA article reiterates that medical conditions in our kinfolk matter. The researchers found that the risk of ASD was 10-fold higher in siblings of ASD patients. And though the risk of ASD lessened as "genetic relatedness declined," there persisted a 2-fold increased risk in cousins of ASD patients.

Clint Eastwood once starred in a movie called **The Good, The Bad and The Ugly**. Perhaps the same relates to our genetic inheritance. However, you should realize that while you may inherit a predilection for a problem, disease is not an inevitability. Science can aid us by identifying potential problems and reducing disease through focused screening and preventive therapies.

So pay attention to your family's medical history and your own health risks. Don't surrender common sense to political correctness. And don't marry your cousin, or your kids may look like Uncle Jack.

We tend to take the natural processes of life for granted. I don't think about breathing or even sleeping very often because they are under the control of subconscious areas of my brain. Actually, patients not infrequently consult me about "breathlessness." Of course shortness of breath can be caused by heart failure and other serious problems, but commonly it's caused by anxiety, which often manifests as breathlessness and excessive "sighing." And most of the time I sleep fine if I just let my nervous system do what it is designed to do, and let go of the cares of the world. Admittedly, that's sometimes easier to say than to do these days.

Everyone has a mother, who once was pregnant and then gave us life through birth. Scientists continue to study the phenomenon of life and even strive to create life by organizing its building blocks. I'm not talking about test tube babies where a human egg is injected with human sperm and the resulting fertilized zygote is then implanted into a woman's womb or uterus. Scientists have not been able to create life, perhaps because we don't have the technology. I would argue that we lack the maturity to handle the implications of this feat. And maybe we are not intended to create life outside of natural processes.

I believe we sometimes take pregnancy for granted. I maintain that it takes almost nothing to father a child, but much more to carry a baby to term and deliver the child into the world. And, it takes even greater efforts to be a parent and raise a child to independence.

I'm certainly not an obstetrician/gynecologist. However, I am an internist who remains fascinated by the intricacies of life and its mechanisms. Recently, an essay in the New England Journal of Medicine (NEJM) caught my eye because it purported to explain a great mystery of why pregnant women go into labor. I've often pondered this question and so have many other scientists. We may be closer to the answer.

Pregnancy is a natural process and yet, why does a mother's immune system not attack and destroy the baby in her uterus? The uterine placenta is the organ through which the baby is provided nourishment and oxygen from the mother. Within the placenta a baby's blood vessels are juxtaposed to the mother's and inevitably their blood streams and immune systems co-mingle.

One reason the baby is not attacked is that pregnancy is a state of "altered immunity." The mother's body "tolerates" the baby even though the child is genetically different, possessing both the mother's and the father's DNA. If you receive an organ transplant you must take immune system suppressing drugs for the rest of your life or the organ will be attacked by the host's immune system and destroyed. This is called "rejection" and is a dreaded complication of transplantation which can result in death. And yet the baby lives and grows because the mother's immune system *tolerates* this different person inside her womb, at least until *parturition*.

The altered state of immunity in pregnancy has other implications. Pregnant women are at an increased risk of infections including influenza virus. I once treated a pregnant woman who developed an infection with an unusual bacterium called listeria. The bacterium was acquired through the ingestion of feta cheese which traditionally was made from unpasteurized goats' milk. Feta cheese now is safe if purchased in a supermarket and made from pasteurized milk. Certain French cheeses like Brie and Camembert should be avoided in pregnancy as well as raw seafood like sushi and raw oysters. Appropriate vaccinations for measles and influenza are also advisable.

The NEJM article is mechanistic and arcane, but offers clues to explain labor and child birth. Multiple researchers have shown that as pregnancy progresses levels of fetal (baby) DNA rise in the mother's blood stream. Interestingly, this DNA circulates outside of cells in a "free" state. It is thought that the DNA is released from the maturing or aging placenta. The rising levels of fetal DNA stimulate receptors on white blood cells and activate an inflammatory process modulated by signaling proteins called cytokines. Together the balanced inflammatory process softens the cervix allowing dilation, and produces uterine contractions, membrane rupture (water breaking) and parturition or childbirth.

Few would challenge the notion that men and women are different. It was my grandson Oakley who reminded me of the differences between boys and girls. Becky and I were blessed with two healthy girls who exuded "sugar and spice and everything nice." My mother had three boys and swears to this day that books would fly off a shelf as her boys entered a room. And the differences of the sexes become even more obvious at puberty and beyond. As a side bar, did you realize that all of us are female in the womb until sex hormones begin to be produced and cause differentiation of the sexes?

I am a rational man, so I suspect it's my genes at work that cause me to see a pregnant woman as beautiful. Women find this observation unfathomable because they perceive themselves as bloated when pregnant. While it can be said that a pregnant woman's body is not beautiful by "runway standards," it was Plato who observed that "beauty lies in the eyes of the beholder." (And Plato was no shabby observer.)

July is blackberry picking time in our part of the world and is ordinarily solitary work. Consequently, a dense patch of berries affords a contemplative time for reflection. One of my favorite books is **Pilgrim at Tinker Creek** by Annie Dillard. This modern-day Thoreau at her Walden Pond observed that "nature is profligate." I see what she means as thousands of berries are produced with the hopes that a few survive to produce more fruit.

By nature men are somewhat like blackberries and dandelions. All are profligate, though reason and a good woman have civilized this man. Evolution demands more of a woman who must choose the best for her consort. Maurice Chevalier said it best, "Thank God for little girls" who grow up to bring life into the world and Grace to their men.

Babies require a lot of work, even for grandparents. I know this because my wife keeps our grandson, Oakley, during the week and I help on Wednesday afternoons. I marvel at Becky's patience and expertise. The half-life of medical information is said to be twenty years. Perhaps the same is true with baby-knowledge because I seem to have forgotten a lot since my girls were tiny, thirty years ago. I recently asked Becky why Oakley tries to put everything in his mouth. She answered in her usual graceful manner reminding me that a baby's mouth is very sensitive, so naturally they use it to test the world around them.

My CBE (continuing baby education instead of continuing medical education) will continue this weekend as we fly to San Diego for a family wedding. We're even preparing goodie bags for the journey, but not for us; the treats are for our fellow travelers on the plane who may be sitting near "The Oakes." A crying baby on a cross country airplane trip can be tough and might provoke a Halloween trick at this time of year. I'm concerned that we'll be flying across three time zones as well as ending Daylight Savings Time this weekend. I have learned over the last six months that you don't mess with a baby's schedule. I may need one of those goodie bags before the weekend is over.

Our trip and Oakley's napping/feeding schedule got me to thinking about travel medicine which has evolved into the specialty called **emporiatrics**. This discipline deals with the complexities of travel and travel safety. These days Americans think nothing of jumping on a plane and flying to the ends of the earth. One of my proverbial sayings is, "Get on a plane, rent a car, and you can see the world." However, another Ferg-ism is "Getting sick is bad, but being sick far from home is even worse."

Oakley doesn't worry about what he puts in his mouth, but you should. Consideration of food preparation and water safety is very important when traveling. Having a Coke on the rocks may sound wonderful in the Guatemalan heat, but I don't recommend it! I once got a tainted cup of hot coffee in the Guatemala City Airport that I paid dearly for over the next several days.

Did you know that the cabins of airplanes are only pressurized to 6000-8000 feet? In other words, if you have serious heart or lung disease you may need supplemental oxygen just as if you had driven to the top of Pike's Peak. Prolonged sitting is also problematic with long plane flights, especially in the cramped coach class. I advise patients to wiggle their toes, get up and walk around, and do deep knee bends in the airplane galley while waiting for the bathroom to clear. This helps to compress the veins in the legs and to prevent blood clots. People at high risk of blood clots can use medications for prevention, but these drugs are tricky to use and expensive. Obviously this issue should be discussed with your doctor.

Not infrequently patients call me for a prescription to prevent motion sickness while they're on a cruise. However, they rarely consider the side effects of the sea sickness patch. Often patients ask me for an antibiotic "in case of a respiratory infection" (usually viral) or for diarrhea, but don't consider that antibiotics often cause diarrhea or that the bacteria of sinus infections are entirely different than those that produce Montezuma's revenge or the Delhi-belly. Folks, there is no such thing as an antibiotic that fits all needs.

The Health Department is often used as a resource by travelers. They do have standard vaccines like tetanus and diphtheria boosters that are advisable every ten years. And they have exotic vaccines and protocols to administer them. However, I recommend that you see your doctor to discuss where you're going, what you'll be doing, and preventive measures that are most appropriate for you. An example emphasizes my point: Hepatitis B is endemic (common) in Southeast Asia. Should all travelers to this region get hepatitis B vaccinations which require a series of three shots over six months? I don't think this is wise if your travel is going to be short or to developed areas like Tokyo, providing you're not planning to get a tattoo or to be intimate with the locals.

Every year people travel to foreign countries without considering malaria prophylaxis. As a result they put themselves at risk for malaria from mosquito bites. West Nile virus and Dengue fever are also spread by mosquitoes. Dengue is endemic in the Caribbean and carries the colorful and descriptive moniker "break back fever." Obviously, protective clothing and mosquito repellants such as DEET are preferable to a *breaking back*.

People often ask me for sleeping pills when they travel. I had a patient who passed out in a airplane galley after two high balls and then popped an Ambien sleeping pill, so I'm pretty sensitive to these requests. Some years ago Becky and I made the journey to Australia. It's a tough trip and I believe it should probably be made sedated! We left Knoxville at 4 PM on a Thursday and landed in Sydney at 8 AM Saturday (we did cross the International Date Line). I tried to calculate how and when to take melatonin to reset my internal clock as we traveled to the other side and to the bottom of the world. The charts and calculations flummoxed me and I'm not sure anything helped except being younger than I am now. After personal and professional study, I believe the best method to become acclimated is to adopt the sleep/wake cycle of your destination.

Though precautions are advisable, travel is still wonderful and I say, "Bon voyage!" But see your travel-sensitive doctor first.

Have you ever wondered why the doctor thumps on your stomach, listens with his stethoscope over your neck and groin, or why he takes that little hammer and raps on your knees? Is he just trying to torment you when he strokes the bottom of your foot with that darn hammer or presses a tuning fork to your big toe, sending vibrations to your teeth? Remember Ferguson's Rule # 3: there is a reason for things. So, sit down with a cup of coffee and I'll explain a bit of the mystery and the applied science of clinical medicine.

Doctors go to medical school to learn the theory of disease or what we call pathology. However, before we learn about disease we are taught how the body functions and what is normal. I equate this with a mechanic who knows about car engines, what goes wrong, and how to diagnose the problem. I love the old Andy Griffith show and its characters. Goober was the cousin of Gomer Pyle and a first-rate car mechanic. I love the episode where Goober is supposed to be minding the courthouse, but can't resist working on a friend's car inside the courthouse!

As medical school juniors, would-be doctors begin to see patients with supervision and learn to examine the body to develop, excuse the pun, a feeling for what is normal. There is no information in a book comparable to the experience of mashing on several hundred bellies. The Internship and Residency training period after medical school is the next level of training with increasing responsibility until you are finally *ready* to solo. It's a daunting experience to sit down across from your first patient and ask her, "How can I help you, *Mrs. Jones?*" You then realize the huge responsibility she has entrusted to you. We doctors are trained to listen, to ask questions, to examine and then to come up with a diagnosis and advice. So let's think about the doctor visit and how it works.

Why do doctors ask you to fill out those personal history forms, after you've worn your pencil to a nub filling out insurance and general information forms? No, it's not because the doctor is lazy; it's to prompt your memory similar to priming a pump. I learned long ago that the second time a person is asked a medical question the answer is more accurate after reflection. You can actually ask the same question too many times and influence the answer. Patience is a virtue; so help your doctor help you. I like to think that my patients and I are a team working together.

After the doctor interviews you an examination follows. The vascular system, which includes the heart, lungs and blood vessels, is a good place to start. The vital signs of heart rate, blood pressure, and respiratory are simple inexpensive measurements of health. Many doctors now include pulse oximetry (a reflection of oxygen in the circulation as a fourth vital sign. You may be surprised to learn that in my career what is considered ideal or *normal* blood pressure has become lower and lower. Science has proven that a blood pressure of 100/60 is better than one of 120/80, and this level is healthier than 150/100. I found it shocking to learn that Franklin D. Roosevelt had a blood pressure of 300/120 late in his life. It was thought at that time that a high blood pressure was needed to force blood through narrow arteries constricted by fatty plaque, somewhat analogous to rust in old pipes. We now know that hypertension accelerates vascular disease and his hypertension undoubtedly contributed to FDR's fatal stroke. I often tell patients that "the questions never change, just the answers." It will probably always be that way.

(This essay first appeared in two parts. The conclusion follows.)

Recall that last week we were discussing blood pressure and the disease hypertension. There is a difference between an elevated blood pressure that can be caused by, for instance, stress or pain, and the sustained elevation of blood pressure we call hypertension. Consider this the next time your blood pressure is checked; for every 20mm increment of the systolic blood pressure (the top number) or 10mm increase of the bottom (diastolic) blood pressure, your risk of cardiovascular disease doubles. This is powerful information that is obtained from a simple low-tech measurement. Given the ease of measuring blood pressure, I believe it should be checked *every* time you see a doctor, even your dermatologist! How's that for controversy?

As I exam the cardiovascular system, I carefully listen to the heart and the lungs with my stethoscope – another useful low-tech instrument. But listening to the heart and lungs goes far beyond the examination. Research shows that patients believe their doctor cares more about them when they are examined, rather than just evaluated across the exam room. I've led a half-dozen foreign medical missions in Central America and I insisted that every patient's heart and lungs be listened to by our doctors. It promotes the notion of care, and is good medicine as well.

I also carefully listen over the arteries of the neck, the abdomen, and the groin area. A whooshing sound of turbulence blood flow is a marker of vascular disease. Have you ever sat by a *roaring* stream and thought about the noise that the water makes as it tumbles over a rock? Similarly, turbulent blood flow in a diseased artery – called a bruit by doctors – can be heard with a stethoscope and is an important sign of vascular disease. Likewise, an enlarged aorta in the abdomen and diminished arterial pulses in the feet are also important clues of cardiovascular disease and should prompt additional studies such as measurement of cholesterol, glucose measurement, and arterial ultrasound testing.

In the abdomen I check the liver and gallbladder which are just under your right lower rib cage. A measure of their size can be estimated by gently feeling and then thumping (we call it percussion) over the ribs and abdomen. The thumping produces slightly different notes over the organs than over the lower chest and lungs. This can be translated to size – perhaps not as accurate as a CAT scan, but a lot cheaper and without radiation exposure.

Everyone is familiar with the reflex hammer and having your knee reflexes tested. But, did you realize that this tapping is a test for nerve disease? And did you know that a brain tumor or a stroke can be detected by stroking the bottom of your foot with the hammer? We doctors don't rub your sole to torment you or to see if you're ticklish! Likewise, degenerative changes of the spinal cord can be detected by testing your toes with a tuning fork. There are of course more sophisticated tests available, but all care begins with a careful history and a thorough examination. Even looking at the skin and nails can give the trained eye important clues to a person's health. Even a simple face-to-face interview affords me with a wealth of information about a patient's physical and emotional health. This is why phone care is often discouraged.

I was taught in medical school that 90% of a diagnosis is made from the history and physical examination. When I was a younger doctor I questioned this assertion. I wanted a CAT scan more than a stethoscope's findings. I have come full circle now and trust my clinical skills more and more. My observation skills have served me well in the mountains of Guatemala. I don't want to throw out technology, but I want to use it with discretion and wisdom and never to replace a caring touch. Isn't that what it's all about?

Laughter is Good Medicine - May 11, 2011

"She is clothed with strength and dignity; she can laugh at the days to come."
Proverbs 31:25

I haven't laughed out loud in a while. You know, those laughs that come from your toes and make your eyes water; those laughs which seem to choke off your breath and make you beg for mercy.

Scientists say that animals laugh. I've never observed my dog Jack laughing, though he does smile at me. I find the claim that primates laugh more plausible, even though I've never observed the phenomenon. I'll concede the point to experts because I've never seen Moscow either, and yet I believe it exists from the observation of others. At some level you have to accept things on faith. Therefore, even though I don't spend a lot of time at our wonderful zoo, I'll accept the fact that animals exhibit this otherwise human vocalization we call laughter.

An expert in laughter believes that laughing must have been one of the earliest forms of human communication. Along with smiling, it is thought that laughter evolved as nuanced communication in social groups to clarify one's intentions. I suspect you'd be less wary of a person laughing heartily than someone approaching you with a frown and a club in his hand.

I find laughter fascinating. Have you ever wondered why a comedian like Seinfeld has a *warm up* act? I'll bet most of us have observed the phenomena of *infectious laughter*, where comedy builds on itself. I believe this is why laugh tracks are played with sitcoms. And I think the same philosophy holds with warm up acts at music concerts. The warm up primes the pump, so to speak.

The most common cause of laughter is a *funny* story or picture. Mark Twain once observed that comedy is the highest art-form. He may be right because I'd wager that most of us have experienced an otherwise funny story told at an inappropriate time or with the wrong group setting that falls flat on its face. Timing with storytelling or comedy is crucial, observe experts. Some believe that laughter serves as an emotional balance to stress. Well, I've witnessed emotional giggles, but not guffaws!

Researchers at the University of Maryland Medical Center have demonstrated that laughter causes blood vessels in the brain to dilate from the release of nitric oxide and endorphins. Endorphins are very potent morphine-like chemicals that modulate pain and stress responses, and may be the cause of the "runner's high" observed by joggers. Nitric oxide regulates blood flow in all vascular beds, even blood vessels in the heart. Perhaps laughter is good for your health, though I'll warn you to be careful around my wife. Trying to provoke laughter with a tickle will produce a violent response and may lead to serious injury from flying elbows and knees. My Becky says tickling t'aint welcome.

It's amazing that such a basic human function as laughter is so poorly understood. I came to the same conclusion in a Focus essay about dreams last year. Even philosophers have weighed in on laughter. Sigmund Freud held to the so called **relief theory,** where laughing releases "psychic energy" as a coping mechanism. Friedrich Nietzsche once said that laughter is a response to existential loneliness. I think that's just pure c**p.

It's been tough for me lately due to all the changes in my world. The economy is in the tank, "wars and rumors of wars" are everywhere, the governmental intrusion into medical care and even the examination room, and now the challenge of organizing a new medical practice arrangement. Long ago my wife gave me a picture and signed it, "Above, beyond, and through it all, I love you." I read this often, especially when I'm in danger of being overwhelmed. The Teacher who wrote the Proverbs understood the value of a good woman and life partner; and she makes me laugh!

So tonight I'll celebrate my 60th birthday with my beautiful wife and my family. We'll talk and eat, drink some wine and enjoy each other's company. Hopefully, we'll tell a few tall tales and laugh. The doctor needs this sabbatical from the cares of the world.

So, here's to life and laughter and happy-ever-afters!

Conflagration - August 8, 2011

I stood among the giant redwoods, and a sense of awe came upon me. There is a reverential quietness in this primeval forest of redwoods nestled along the California coastline just north of San Francisco. Nature's special micro climate and the conservationist wisdom of man preserve this special place named after the naturalist John Muir.

If you've never been to Muir Woods you must put it on your *bucket list*. The giant redwoods tower above visitors and form a cathedral without equal. This special place evokes words of scripture and the hymn, "Surely the presence of the Lord is in this place."

As Becky and I walked in quiet contemplation we would occasionally pause and listen as park rangers gave nuanced details of the forest. One startling fact emerged that explained the charred bases of the redwoods and the dearth of underbrush so common in our eastern forests. The ranger said that the redwood cones, with their precious seeds, open only when a fire burns through the forest and removes the cloying underbrush that would otherwise limit sunlight and choke out the tiny saplings. The charred bark of the giants was a testament to fires over the eons and nature's design.

In 1988 a huge fire engulfed Yellowstone Park burning more than a million acres of this national treasure. It was thought that Yellowstone was gone and would never recover. The hubris of man never fails to astound me, and the experts were again proved wrong. The forest recovered and is now better than ever. The entire fire suppression policy which allowed decades of brush to accumulate and provided fuel for inevitable fires was revamped. Now, controlled burning to remove underbrush is the modus operandi of forest management experts.

Humans are subject to the fires of fever. After my internal medicine training I considered doing a fellowship in infectious disease, which the Chinese represent with a symbol which means *hot disease*. I decided to stay with internal medicine, and later passed my boards in Geriatrics which is now recognized as a subspecialty of internal medicine.

I've always been intrigued by fever. The measurement of temperature is one of the vital signs. Too often patients don't check their temperature; I assure you it is an important diagnostic clue and a measure of illness. I once read a study that compared temperature, patient age, and the probability of serious disease. It turns out that a temperature of 101° Fahrenheit in a patient over sixty years old indicates a serious problem with a 90% probability. Folks, this is powerful information. Similar temperature elevations in younger adults and children have less prognostic import.

You might ask why your body produces fever when it's sick. It turns out that fever develops in the presence of inflammation which releases chemical messengers called cytokines. These proteins rev up the immune system and mobilize our defenses to combat invasion by microorganisms. Interestingly, bacteria require iron to multiply yet can't store this necessary element, and are therefore dependent on the host to supply their needs. Fever suppresses iron release from storage sites in our bodies, and the lower circulating iron levels deprive invading bacteria of a crucial growth factor.

The equivalent of a fire now burns uncontrolled in our country, and I'm worried. A friend of mine says that worry is a poor testament of faith. Perhaps he's right. Perhaps I shouldn't worry about the barely civil war that is consuming our land. But how does one not care? I'm just not made that way. It would be easier if I was a Pollyanna, but I'm not.

So as I try each day to do my best I turn to the lessons of nature and scripture and experience to find my way. Perhaps it's time for a great fire to burn away the underbrush that has accumulated over the decades in forest America. Perhaps new saplings of freedom will germinate and flourish when given the opportunity. I worry about the innocents in this war against the misguided philosophies which produced this mess. However, nature teaches us that life isn't necessarily fair. I believe there is a delicate balance between giving someone a hand up or a hand out. The latter stifles and keeps people in slavery.

The phoenix called America will arise anew; I have faith. It will be tough in the coming years, but we'll be OK if we do our best and our duty, and "keep looking up." The State is not the answer; it is the Spirit.

The Sound of Rain - September 12, 2011

I'm resting on this Labor Day, and I need it. My wife, Becky has just about worked me to death over the previous two days. Our newest project, Thistle Farm, a sort of "Green Acres" is a big one, as if our lives weren't already full. The plan was for a third day of bush hogging, but thankfully The Lord sent rain and I can sit with my thoughts and rest my bones.

Usually I write my stories on Wednesday, but as I sat on the porch this morning the sound of rain caught my attention, and *that's when the story began.* You realize that falling rain makes no sound; the noise is generated when tens of thousands of leaves are struck with wet missiles. It's fascinating how similar this sound compares to water rushing over rocks in a mountain stream. There's a stream above Gatlinburg called the Roaring Forks which captures this imagery quite well.

As a doctor I'm always searching for gurgling noises in the arteries of my patients which doctors call *bruits.* We all know that deep water runs silently, but when it tumbles over rocks it roars. Similarly, blood flowing through smooth arteries is not restricted and moves silently. However, when an obstruction develops, because of a build-up of fatty deposits called plaque, turbulence is produced which can be heard with a stethoscope placed over the arteries in the neck, abdomen, and groin areas. Turbulent blood flow from a damaged heart valve causes a similar sound doctors refer to as a heart murmur. This sounds like you're repeatedly shushing someone with a "shhh, shhh, shhh."

I actually like rain, as long as it's less than forty days and nights, or rain that occurs on your daughter's garden wedding day. Rain often slows the pace of life, and I welcome that interlude. It would be nice to control the weather and make it rain in Texas and Oklahoma where there is an historic drought. The people in New England I'm sure would have no problem sharing some of hurricane Irene's recent excess with their western neighbors. Weather control is a frequent storyline in science fiction genre, but we currently don't have the technology or the wisdom to tamper with the forces of nature. We even have difficulty predicting whether it will rain this evening.

I read today of an experiment supported by the Royal Academy and funded by the British government. They propose to float a helium balloon the size of a soccer field into the stratosphere, tethered to the ground by a hose, to spray water into the upper atmosphere to deflect the sun's heat and reduce global warming. Folks, I'm not making this up; the foolishness and hubris of man seems alive and well in England and Al-Gore.

The world is complex and is always changing. It was miserably hot and humid last week and now it's not. Seventy million years ago the CO2 content in the atmosphere was 0.1% as compared to today's 0.04%. The world was much warmer then, the vegetation was lusher due to the abundant CO2, and an inland sea extended from our Gulf of Mexico into Tennessee. As boys, my brothers and I found large fossilized snails from the Paleozoic era in our back yard. These snails had once crawled on that ancient sea floor.

If you've never been to Niagara Falls, you must add it to your bucket list. The power and majesty of the Niagara River tumbling over the rock escarpment is majestic and humbling. But more amazing is the realization that 70 thousand years ago the ice pack at Niagara Falls was one mile deep because the Earth was in a glacial period. In fact, it was the glaciers that gouged out the Great Lakes basin, and when the Earth began to warm again (twelve thousand years ago) the melting ice filled Lake Superior to a depth of 1,000 feet.

We humans can't be blamed for using our observational skills to try and figure things out. Unfortunately, we have trouble looking beyond our immediate and limited horizons. It's obvious that it's hot right now, but it's supposed to be because it's late summer.

About a year ago I read a story by a journalist who researched the media's cyclical hype of the weather over the last 100 years. He found that there were dire warnings of global cooling in the late 1800's, followed by equally dire warnings of global warming in the 1930s. We all remember that it was colder in the 1970s which *Time*, *Look*, and other major news periodicals called another **Little Ice Age** – after its namesake of 1550 to 1850. This of course came after the medieval warming period during which the Vikings established colonies in __Green__land, for heaven's sake.

The hype now is anthropogenic or man-made global warming which they now call *climate change* perhaps because there hasn't been any warming for over a decade. And there wasn't any man-made CO2 when Lief Ericson was planting grape vines in Greenland. My point is to look beyond what the media and the politicians are saying and consider *why* they're saying such and such. I'll admit I'm a skeptic, and I don't believe much of anything Al-Gore says; after all he's a politician.

No, my title is not a typo. Nor am I referring to Google, the internet search engine, or a Gothic gargoyle. These days we are bombarded with information and often presented with numbers that stagger the mind. I remember when a millionaire was someone like Thurston Howell III on Gilligan's Island. I've never known anyone like Thurston or Lovey.

Now, the wealthiest have **billions** of dollars instead of millions. I once read that the definition of being rich is when your money works for you rather than you working for your money. However, billionaires like Warren Buffett and Bill Gates are pikers when compared to Uncle Sam, who collects and spends **trillions** of dollars every year. Unfortunately, our Uncle spends more than we have in our pockets and has run up a ruinous debt of more than 16 trillion dollars.

About ten years ago I located my high school chemistry and physics teacher to thank him for my medical career. His method for balancing chemical equations and handling large numbers enabled me to do well enough in college to be accepted into medical school. Most of us recall someone who made a difference in our lives. It was Mr. Hardin at West High School who made a difference for me, and I told him so as I shook his hand.

A billion is a thousand million, and a trillion is a thousand billion. It's easier to think of these big numbers using powers of 10. As an example, a trillion is 1 followed by twelve zeros, and it's easier to represent this big number as 10^{12}, where the superscript represents the number of zeros. It's a necessity to use this system of representation when you try to conceptualize the data collection system our government is developing in Bluffdale, Utah.

This two billion dollar project will be fully operational in September 2013. I remember the Star Wars movie when Darth Vader was told the Death Star was likewise "fully operational." The government's storage facility will have a capacity of storing a **septillion** bytes of data. This staggering number is also known as a **yottabyte** – not to be confused with Yoda the Jedi Knight.

Computer buffs casually speak of **gigabytes** of hard drive memory. The rest of us refer to this amount of storage capacity as a billion. A **terabyte** is a trillion (1000 billion) pieces of data that can be carried on a flash drive no larger than you pinky finger, and carried in your pocket to Russia. Apparently, NSA's (National Security Agency) Edward Snowden did just that and eloped to Hong Kong before moving to Moscow. However, 10^{12} pieces of data pale by comparison to an **exabyte** or 10^{18} pieces of data. It has been estimated that all human knowledge can be stored in five exabytes. NSA's Bluffdale facility will have yottabyte (10^{24})

capacity or a million exabytes. One wonders why the NSA needs one million times the storage capacity of all human knowledge. Our "spooks" say that their *Meta-data-mining* project called PRISM is necessary for our safety. Others feel this dragnet is an infringement of our privacy and a violation of the Constitution's Fourth Amendment intended to limit the government's power to search through our lives.

I've read that our Milky Way galaxy has approximately 300 billion stars, or thirty times the number of brain cells between our ears. Some of us get a lot done with those brain cells. But even this large number is eclipsed by the 30 trillion cells in the human body, a number that is a 1000 times the stars in the Milky Way. But don't focus on our stellar neighbor; look up and beyond. There are more than 100 billion galaxies in the Universe, resulting in 10^{22} stars in the Creation. More stars than there are grains of sand on all the beaches of the world. God creates beyond exabytes!

A friend of mine maintains that humans think in templates or patterns or pictures. I already knew a lot of things about my dog Jack before we ever brought him home because I know about dogs. They have four legs, excellent hearing and smell, and poorer eyesight than a human. I knew about Jack because of the canine template. Perhaps other thoughtful beings on other planets circling other suns think differently. We may never know because the Universe is so vast, and we are constrained by the cosmological speed limit of light. Imagine riding on the fastest space vehicle man has ever built and traveling to our Sun's closest neighbor. You would arrive at Alpha Centauri in 70,000 (70×10^3) years.

I've come to the point in life where I know what's right. This may sound like hubris, when actually it's a statement of fundamental and foundational principles which define my being. It doesn't mean I've stopped listening and learning, or sifting through the megabytes (millions) of data that swirl around me. To stop learning would be, for me, to die. Last week I mentioned the book **How Should We Then Live?** This is where I am now in my contemplation. Schaeffer proffers four directives for these difficult times and I concur: the Bible is the inspired word of God; we need a relationship with the Creator; we must speak the truth; and we must have compassion for the confused and the lost.

I've found that fundamental truths are fewer in number than the world's sometimes confusing data. I have a friend who's a computer programmer and believes humans think in multiples of ten because we have ten fingers. He says using a base eight system would make things easier for computer programmers. I'll mention that to the Master when I see Him. I also want to ask about the limits of knowledge and if the hypothetical **googol: 10^{100}** really exists.

It's hard not to write about something on your mind or something that's in your body. I have a family history of colon and prostate cancer and as a result my doctors have their way with me on a regular basis.

I no longer watch NBC because of its bias, but as I was flipping channels I learned that Matt Lauer and Al Roker were to get prostate cancer screening tests during their morning TV show. By the titillating tone of the advertisement, I assumed their screening test wasn't a PSA (prostate specific antigen) blood test. After all, it was on the Today show that Katie Couric had her first colonoscopy. I suspect the boys were to have the ever so popular DRE or digital rectal exam. Recently, I similarly assumed the position and steeled myself for the probing. My doctor said, "Jim, I'm sorry." Glancing over my left shoulder and through gritted teeth, I managed a growl, "Doc, you're not as sorry as I am."

Cancer screening is an important aspect of medical care and is a focus of the Annual Wellness Visit now mandated by Obamacare. Never mind that competent physicians have always advised their patients of appropriate cancer screening tests as they monitored and treated other conditions at a fraction of the cost now expended. We now have an additional expensive layer of bureaucracy to organize screening tests that our children and their children will be forced to repay.

Most of my readers understand that a colonoscopy is the procedure of choice to screen for colon cancer, and the biggest hurdle of the "scope" is the prep. By the time the prep has spent the night scrubbing your insides, the worst is over and the examination is a snap. I have to admit that my doctor's purgative protocol was a big improvement over preps I've endured with previous examinations. In my personal experience the worst is the "gallon jug" purgative regimen. One of my gastrointestinal colleagues admitted to me that after he experienced the gallon-jug prep for his colonoscopy he no longer uses it with his patients.

I believe we are too quick to complain and slow to compliment those who do a good job. The staff at Fort Sanders Hospital took good care of me and I told them so. And I survived my scope with a good report. Years ago Demerol and Versed were given as sedation for colonoscopy examinations. Propofol is the sedating drug used these days. I've had both regimens and Propofol is better as long as it is used by professionals in a controlled situation. You may remember that Propofol was the drug used by Michael Jackson's doctor to put him to sleep every night. Jackson died and the doctor went to jail. I went to sleep in ten seconds and awakened twenty-five minutes later with only minimal side effects. Case in point, I'm writing this essay after my procedure and sedation.

I've written before that threes resonate with me. I'm a Trinitarian at heart and Becky says I can always find three options in most situations. I believe two choices aren't enough, and four is too many. One option is not a choice, but three is just about right!

A couple of weeks ago I wrote about *three* patients who had fallen. Two had broken hips and a third a fractured pelvis. This week it seems that breast cancer is unfortunately the diagnosis in *three* of my patients. Sometimes older ladies resist going for mammography or a doctor's examinations. That is a mistake because breast cancer risk doesn't decline as you get older. However, a mammogram isn't enough. Three years ago an eighty-eight year old lady came to me as a new patient. She reported two hospitalizations in the previous six months. She told me that none of the numerous doctors who cared for her examined her breasts. I did so and she had breast cancer. She is alive today because of a careful examination and curative surgery.

No test is perfect. If designed for screening purposes a test needs to be very sensitive, and we have to accept some false positives. On the other hand, some tests are designed to be very specific and would be poor screening procedures because many subtle abnormalities might be overlooked. The bottom line is that you and your doctor are a team and should be the ones who decide what is best for you. This should not be done by an insurance company or a politically motivated President.

Screening tests help, but most of us know what we should do to stay healthy; it's not rocket science. We shouldn't use tobacco or overeat. We should exercise and wear seat belts. Diseases that run in your family matter and influence healthcare decisions, even screening tests. Illicit drugs kill the soul and the body. The Spirit is foundational. William Penn, the founder of the Pennsylvania colony said three hundred years ago, "Those who will not be ruled by God will be ruled by tyrants." Mr. Penn understood that Spirit trumps State.

As a conservative I believe in the freedom of choice, but I accept the consequences of those choices. If you use street drugs and develop health problems you should be rescued once and offered rehab. If you refuse then tough love must reign and you will have to go to the end of the line for any additional help in a world of limited resources. Jesus said that the "poor will always be with you." I believe this applies to the poor in spirit as well as imperfect health and limited abilities.

Our erstwhile President crows about equality, though divides us further in his speeches and policies. Unfortunately, equality is a utopian concept. I recognize that I will never be as good a person as my wife who is one of the few genuinely good people I have encountered. However, in a Republic we are supposed to have equal opportunity under the law. But how can we trust a man or his minions who repeatedly violate the fundamental procedures of the Constitution and its laws?

What kind of animal fouls its own nest? I thought about this as I gazed at the discarded trash bags thrown into my yard. I try to walk a couple of miles at least three times a week, and I often carry a small trash bag to pick up litter in the neighborhood. A young man who lives down the street from us, sporting Rastafarian dreadlocks, once stopped to ask Becky and me what we were doing. I told him we were picking up trash while we walked and invited him to join us. He looked at me perplexed and never returned to participate in our community clean up.

However, the multiple trash bags of litter strewn through our neighborhood this time represented an escalation of simple littering. Perhaps these *creatures of the hood* were marking their new territory, as do animals, or just had a callous disregard of others and the environment. As I worked to clean up the mess I wondered if this was another example of the further devolution of morality in our culture.

Years ago Becky published an essay in *Newsweek Magazine* when that periodical was actually read and was worth millions of dollars instead of its sale price of $1 in 2010. Her essay was about petty crimes that go unpunished and then escalate to more serious ones – somewhat analogous to our current US foreign policy. My Kroger plastic bags have always been adequate for the occasional beer bottle or Sonic Styrofoam cup thrown along our roadside. It took gloves, my truck and multiple trash bags to clean up the scat that these devolved criminals dropped not fifty feet from the Knox County road sign threatening a fine of $1000 for littering. The perpetrators probably feel safe because our constables are often focused on more heinous crimes these days.

In medicine we often deal with multilevel impoverishment. There are people who are financially poor. There are people who are intellectually challenged or ill-educated and often duped by our perverse media. And there are people who, as Jesus described in his Sermon on the Mount, are poor in spirit. Renunciation of a higher power and substituting the *law of the jungle* or the *hood* makes for animalistic behavior. But even animals don't soil their own nests.

Already in the month of September three of my patients went to the emergency room for non-emergencies including a sore pinky toe, a scraped finger and a bug bite. You say that's ridiculous and a misuse of valuable resources, and I say it's common because there's no accountability or consequences of inappropriate behavior. This is not a new phenomenon, but it is escalating. I once asked a woman why she called an ambulance to bring her to the ER where I was working. She told me she didn't have the cab fare to transport her to the hospital so that she could have her IUD removed.

There is a kerfuffle of late regarding Mr. Romney's statement that the 47% (actually 46.4%) of American citizens don't pay any income taxes and would probably favor Mr. Obama in the November election. It doesn't take rocket scientist intellect to concur with candidate Romney's statement. Yet the media and President Obama, on his latest David Letterman gig, were horrified that Romney would state the obvious. Even Republican pundits said that Romney was stupid to tell people the truth.

Many Americans have become impoverished because they focus more on their feelings instead of facts. Did you know that those below the poverty line are affluent by the world's standards? Eighty percent of those below the poverty line have air conditioning, 2/3 have cable TV, 1/2 have a computer, 49% have Internet access, and one in three has a plasma screen TV. As John Adams once said, "Facts are such troublesome things." In an age of information, how can so many be ill-educated, disengaged and deceived? It's called *The Big Lie*. Google it and read of its author and understand that it is being used on you.

I've never been one to think much about the End Times. In fact, the Master once said that anyone who says they know about these issues is an imposter. However, I believe something is happening in our world. The Middle East is in flames. There are "wars and rumors of wars." Even the News Sentinel this week acknowledges our divided country which I published in their paper in 2010 called our **Barely Civil War**. America has turned away from its roots and from "Nature's God" mentioned four times in the Declaration of Independence. How amazing that James Madison and the others who crafted the Constitution in 1789 never mention God. When asked why, Madison said they "just forgot." And so have we.

This election is like no other in our lifetime and perhaps America's history. We are headed for destruction, yet people who no longer relate to facts embrace feelings in slogans such as "Hope and Change" and "Forward." We can still turn away from the brink of bankruptcy, dependency, entitlement, and lack of personal responsibility. And we can again embrace "In God We Trust" and rediscover our roots in 2 Chronicles 7:14. Or, we can end up on the ash heaps of history as so many in the past have done just like Shelley's *Ozymandias*. Puzzled by this reference? Then Google it!

The chief professor of medicine during my internal medicine residency held that all disease was the result of some infectious process. Jesus used hyperbole (exaggerated speech) to get people's attention, and I suspect my professor was doing the same. Because Dr. Stollerman was an expert in infectious diseases and did original investigations of streptococcal infections, such as strep throat and nephritis (kidney inflammation), he was vigilant and felt that germs were the root cause of disease.

We take for granted a functioning immune system until it is damaged by chemotherapy, radiation or by autoimmune diseases like Lupus. Lupus occurs when the immune system dysfunctions and begins to recognize a patient's own blood vessels as alien. The resulting attack produces inflammation in the vessels, a process doctors call vasculitis. A similar immune mechanism occurs in rheumatoid arthritis when the immune system pathologically identifies a person's joints as foreign and attacks them. The resulting pain, swelling, and redness is the result of joint inflammation.

Our immune system consists of white blood cells made in the bone marrow and the lymph glands. These cells produce antibodies that circulate in the bloodstream along with certain white blood cells that regulate immune responses to infection and injury. Cancer specialists (oncologists) often give chemotherapy to combat cancer and hopefully the therapy does more damage to out of control and rapidly growing cancer cells than healthy tissues and the immune system. You may find it surprising, but antibiotics merely support the patient until their marrow recovers from harsh chemotherapy. Inevitably, without bone marrow and immune system recovery after chemo, death ultimately ensues from microbial invasion.

Most of us have read about the atom bombs that were dropped on Hiroshima and Nagasaki to end World War II. As horrible as it seems today, all-out war was then waged not only on military targets, but on civilian populations who supported war industries. However, that was long ago and we've forgotten that many died after the blast from radiation damage to the survivor's bone marrow. The closest modern equivalent is the Chernobyl meltdown in the Ukraine and the Fukushima disaster in Japan. We probably will never learn the number of later deaths from radiation exposure in the Ukraine. Many emergency workers in the Ukraine died from acute exposure as they fought the meltdown generated fires. We do know that the supervisor at the Fukushima plant stayed at his post and ultimately died from acute radiation exposure.

Many of us remember the story of Alexander Fleming who fortuitously discovered penicillin in 1929, ushering in the antibiotic age. Fewer of us know about Ignaz

Simmelweis. This Hungarian physician challenged established thought in 1847 with his proof that the life threatening infections associated with labor and delivery called child-bed fever (puerperal sepsis) could be drastically reduced by doctors washing their hands with a chlorinated lime solution. He was ridiculed and ultimately was committed to an asylum where he died after being beaten by guards shortly after his incarceration. He was ultimately vindicated when Louis Pasteur established the "germ theory." We now take for granted hygienic measures and use hand sanitizers and sterilize the skin before surgery.

I still read multiple medical journals, and recently the New England Journal of Medicine (NEJM) closed the loop for me on the common disease age-related macular degeneration (AMD). My grandmother lost her vision to the "dry" subset of this disease associated with proteinaceous deposits in the retina with atrophy (withering). The "wet" type also has the additional feature of abnormal blood vessels (neovascular) in the retina. These new vascular structures bleed more easily accelerating damage to the delicate retina. Scientific advances have led to therapies that retard growth of these unstable vessels and limit bleeding. Interestingly, when doctors look through the pupil (window) they can directly observe the vascular system and the course of disease.

Researchers have recently discovered a genetic aberration that can lead to dysregulation of the immune system and produce an inflammatory complex in AMD called an inflammasome. This in turn activates components of the inflammatory cascade similar to that seen in gout and another joint problem called pseudogout. I have written previously about inflammatory mechanisms in diseases like Alzheimer's Disease and arteriosclerosis (hardening of the arteries). I find it fascinating that AMD, another disease associated with aging, is also associated with dysregulation of the immune system and inflammation.

The immune system regulates itself through proteins produced by white cells called cytokines. These signaling chemicals enable cells to "talk" to each other and modulate the immune response to foreign invasion or injury. Apparently, congenital genetic defects and those acquired through radiation, chemo or even aging can lead to immune system dysregulation and disease. Perhaps my old professor was, in part, correct. If the skin is damaged allowing bacteria to invade, or if the immune system breaks down, disease results. We now see farther into the mechanisms of disease. At one time we asked the question, "What went wrong?" Now, we ask "why did it go wrong?"

Science explores the universe with what is called reductionism. This is a process where a complex whole is broken down into its component parts in an attempt to understand the whole by comprehending the integral parts.

Yes, we do see farther than we once did, and I suspect this will continue as we strive to learn about our world and explore our purpose. I've been in medicine forty years and it is intriguing to find that complex and seemingly diverse conditions like heart disease, dementia, gout, and AMD may all have a similar etiology. Maybe my old professor was right and these common diseases are all triggered by some obscure viral or other infectious stress on the immune system of a genetically predisposed patient.

The Apostle Paul once observed that we "see dimly as in a mirror." Someday we will see more completely. Until that time I'll keep my eyes open. After all, they are the windows of disease and the soul.

What's In a Name? - December 1, 2014

We don't answer our landline (phone) very much these days because it's usually telemarketers or, most recently, political messages. For Becky and me our iPhones have become our traveling offices and communication centers. I'm not advertising "smart phones," but these personal computers and cell phones are better mousetraps and are truly windows on the world.

However, when the "unidentified" call came in, for some reason, Becky decided to answer our home phone. It was an unusual call and truly from an unidentified caller. There was no heavy breathing, just a series of questions to verify that the caller had reached the right James V. Ferguson. You see, the mystery caller wanted to return a long lost personal keepsake and had only reached our home number through a Google search of Jimmy Ferguson's in Knoxville, Tennessee.

Names are very personal items and not only identify the person, but also, in some ways, describe them. Names were very important in antiquity and often helped define a person. The same philosophy is operative in our friends from Burundi, who I'm happy to report have just passed their American citizenship requirements. They came to America seven years ago as legal refugees from war torn Burundi and Rwanda and had to wait seven years, pay a lot of money and pass citizen examinations to earn their place alongside the rest of us. In their native land their names were given to each child to echo a parent's loving aspirations.

Anthropologists believe Paleolithic man drew pictures on cave walls of the animals they hunted to capture the spirit of their prey. It is thought that these pictographic drawings in Lascaux, France and Altamira, Spain were done to aid the hunter who perhaps needed an edge to be successful in the hunt and thus survive. And because writing had not yet been invented, perhaps stone-age hunters were honoring the spirits of the beasts which would be sacrificed to provide man life-giving sustenance.

The caller wanted to speak with *Jimmy* Ferguson. I have joked with Becky over the years that the only people who call me Jimmy were the ones who knew me before puberty. Though I carry my dad's name, I no longer use Jimmy. And I rarely write "Jr." at the end of my name, now that my dad has passed on, thus ending the confusion. When he was alive I came to use M.D. at the end of my official moniker, though the IRS still knows me as Jr. Perhaps I should call Lois Lerner and clarify this point.

Thanksgiving is a time of family and friends where we celebrate life and blessings, and remember those who made this great country possible. Thanks-giving is just that. It is a time of gathering and tradition. It's a time of feasting and story-telling.

144

In other Focus essays I've spoken of my namesake. My dad was a warrior in WW II; a naval aviator who flew a Dauntless SBD bomber from the bobbing flight deck of the aircraft carrier, Yorktown. He was the patriarch of our family and an architect of tough love. Fortunately, my mother tempered his steel with her loving softness or his boys might have carried scars rather than the enduring lessons of life built on the foundational principles of honor. Growing up, my brothers and I were blessed to have the best of both world views, and this Thanksgiving we are blessed to still have our mother with us.

In recent years we've come to associate negative principles with certain names. Americans have learned what it means to become "Kiffened," after the infamous Lane Kiffen. Just this last week a media person wondered if America has been "Gruberized" by the deceitful Jonathan Gruber, the architect of Obama-care. My dad was honest to a fault and taught us that you are a man of your word or you are nothing.

"Mrs. Ferguson, after talking with you I know I have the right Ferguson family and I need to explain my call. Nearly forty years ago I was in your in-laws' home as a friend of a friend of your husband's brother. (Confused?!) I was loaned Mr. Ferguson's Navy cap, his flight jacket, a flyer's scarf and his Naval Aviator bracelet for a Halloween costume party. I returned everything the next day and went back to ETSU and the rest of my life.

Recently, my Mother passed away and while going through and cleaning her house I found an old box of my swim medals. However, in the bottom of the box was a tarnished bracelet, apparently left absentmindedly in my pants' pocket and found by my Mother while doing my college laundry. The memories came flooding back when I saw the bracelet and that's when I began my internet search to return this keepsake to its rightful owner."

My dad's Naval Aviator bracelet is not a fine piece of jewelry. In fact, I never knew him to wear any adornments other than a ring. It's simple and silver and festooned only with the easily recognizable Naval Aviator Wings emblem. However, on the reverse side there is an inscription which reads, *Jimmy V. Ferguson.*

The inscription was like a time machine drawing me back to my youth and my father's home. The keepsake reminded me of my roots and reconnected me to him. Apparently, as a kid and even as a young adult he was a *Jimmy*. I only knew him as Jim (and, of course, Dad). Now, it seems I have something else in common with Dad besides a feisty temperament. Now, *Jimmy* will always be a name we share and a moniker of the honor he taught me.

And the loop was closed this Thanksgiving as we returned the special bracelet to its rightful owner, my mother, Pat. It is said that we are all a product of our past. We are all thankful and blessed to be the sons and family of *Jimmy* and *Pat*.

A wise man once observed that we all have "gifts differing." We can't all hit a major league fast ball, conceptualize relativity, or provide the nurturing spirit of Mother Teresa. But each of us has unique abilities, and we need to find these and use them. Equality is a postmodern illusion. However, equal *opportunity* under our Constitution is an inalienable right of humans that we must champion.

I'm not a troglodyte as a colleague once jokingly said of my reluctance to embrace electronic medical records. Actually, I use technology and especially computers every day. The iPhone in my pocket is an inseparable extension of my persona and a more powerful computer than any IBM mainframe of the sixties. We're going through a computer upgrade in my medical practice and the challenging adaptation got me thinking about informatics and the Nike slogan. I believe there are striking differences in the way baby boomers like me and the generation Xs and millennials relate to new technology.

Do you consult a map before you go on a trip or read the directions before you begin an assembly? Becky and I do. But, several years ago a thirty-something friend of mine taught me a valuable lesson. I was wondering about a business location and he said, "Why don't you just Google it?" Now I consult the Web dozens of times a day in the care of my patients, to further my education, to find where I'm going as well as satisfying my curiosity.

Neighbors of mine recently decided to redo their kitchen themselves and somehow got one of the home improvement TV shows to chronicle their odyssey. The show opened on the first day of the demolition, and I marveled at their boldness (or foolishness?) as they consulted the Internet on how to begin the demolition. Folks, this is a 21st century mindset. They didn't ruminate over plans or consult experienced contractors, they consulted the Net, and with a crow bar in hand, they forged ahead and just did it. Nike nailed the philosophy of the younger generation.

I'm trying to learn new computer skills, and I've pressed my daughter into service to teach me as I once taught her. The problem is I want to understand what she's doing, and she doesn't really care why she does things; she just plays around with the keys and eventually figures it out. I'm sure some of you have asked your kids or grandkids to program your cell phone with important numbers, or hook up your computer so you can do emails. It seems so easy for these kids who've grown up with techy things. I guess it's in their blood. It's not in mine because I have to stretch myself to keep up. The lesson is to let go; "Feel the Force," as Yoda might say. Don't be afraid to screw up or be intimidated. And by all means don't worry that you'll break "the damn thing." You won't.

Perhaps I'm more *hardwired* now than I once was. When you build a house you have temporary wiring that hangs between the studs where the walls will someday be. You better be sure where you want your electrical outlets because once the walls are up it's very expensive to make changes. To a certain extent our minds are like this electrical simile. We become more hard wired as we get older and it's more difficult to change. However, recent scientific data shows that our brains continue to make new neural connections all our lives. In fact, this is the way we learn. There are neural connections made long ago that enable you to still ride a bike. And I can learn new computer skills or the latest medical advancement.

A friend of mine likes to say, "You're either growing or you're dying," and I believe he's right. I need to keep growing and learning new things and so do you. I believe man (in the generic sense) was meant to work and to serve. Why should we accept retirement at some arbitrary age? My father-in-law taught me a valuable lesson about giving some years ago. He said you should, "Give until it feels good, not until it hurts."

Now, roll up your sleeves, get back to work and "*Just do it!*"

My brother sent me a text saying that our friend had "passed-on." This was not an unexpected announcement since Mitchell was in a Hospice program ending a valiant battle with pancreatic cancer. In forty years of medical care I've only known two patients who have survived this scourge, and unfortunately Mitchell was not the third.

I first met Mitchell on a trek up Mount LeConte. You remember perfect moments, and that beautifully clear October day was a 10. You learn a lot about someone when you labor together or help each other up a mountain. You also learn intimate secrets about a person while sharing a crowded cabin and yelling at him to roll over to stifle his snoring. I said good-bye to Mitchell at his funeral last week on a cold and rainy night so different than when we met on the mountain. Winter temperatures don't plunge as low in our Smoky Mountains as in the Rocky Mountains, but we have what is known as "southern cold" where the cold damp air chills to the bone. I was chilled to the bone this night.

We live in what is called the Bible Belt because a faith perspective is such an important part of our local heritage. I'm glad for these roots, not because I can magically call upon God to fix my problems, but because I trust in something bigger than I can understand. The Proverbist said it best, "Trust in the Lord with all your heart and soul, and not in your own understanding." During Mitchell's funeral service the minister said that a loved one is not lost if you know where they've gone. I'll admit I can't fully comprehend this, but I've come to accept and embrace this perspective. It's a better way to live than existentialism.

We southerners often say that people have "passed-on" instead of saying that they died or passed away. The 16th century humanist Rabelais on his deathbed was purported to have said, "I go to seek a Great...Perhaps." No one knows what happens at death, an experience that none of us can escape. Raymond Moody's book, *Life After Life*, gives us the well-known composite glimpses of near-death experiences which appear to be timeless and cross cultural in their similarities.

My regular readers realize that I love movies, though I recoil at much of the Hollywood culture that so often panders to the basest elements of our society. As an art form movies can nuance stories in a way that books sometimes cannot. I realize that I'm not a *trained* movie critic, but I recently saw the cinema adaptation of Victor Hugo's *Les Miserables*, and it is wondrous. You must go and experience this timeless tale of situational ethics told with marvelous music and evocative acting. While some of the vocals may not be Broadway quality, the storytelling and the passion of the characters are magnificent. At the end, the protagonist Jean Val Jean "passes-on" and is led by the spirit Fantine to the other side of the barricade – truly a remarkable depiction of life after death. And if this whets your appetite, I also recommend *Brainstorm* for another vision of the other side. I believe there is more than we can know and this makes the universe more majestic for me.

I deal with death and dying every day. Doctors want their folks to live long and well. I once told an elderly patient that it was my job to get him to 100 years old and after that it was the Lord's responsibility. Of course I was kidding because my efforts are minimal in the scope of things. I do encourage people to make healthy choices that will maximize their odds of a successful and long life. Some listen and make those tough choices, rewarding the doctor and his patient.

Our mortal bodies will one day cease to function in what we call death. My job is to push death and dying off into the future and, when death is inevitable, help people make the transition as painlessly as possible. There is a saying, "I don't fear death, only the dying." How true this is. I've always wondered why some women have easy labor bringing life into the world and some have it tough. I have the same question at the end of life, where some go to sleep and hopefully awaken in paradise, and some struggle mightily in the transition. The Hospice movement is helpful in this final transition and serves patients as well as their families – and doctors, who sometimes need to let go.

Life is precious at any age, yet the greatest adventure lies ahead of us. Perhaps some may consider this perspective foolish or maudlin. I would argue that those who say there is nothing more than what they can prove or understand deny the wisdom of luminaries such are Plato, Jesus, Augustine, Aquinas, Luther, and Einstein. How limiting and sad this perspective which seems increasingly prevalent in our 21st century.

I heard an interview of an atheist on NPR recently who remains angry and lost twelve years after her husband's death. I thought to myself, the husband wasn't the only person lost. Mitchell's family disagrees with that perspective and because of their faith they can celebrate his life with a quote from Dr. Seuss, "Don't cry because it's over, smile because it happened."

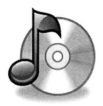

"The Day that UT Died" - May 24, 2010

I hope that Don McLean won't be offended that I thought of his song *American Pie* as "Al-gore" stepped to the podium. Al was in Knoxville to receive his honorary doctorate in Laws and Human Letters in Ecology and Evolutionary Biology from my alma mater. From all the chatter, it's obvious that the debate about Global Warming... uh, Climate Change... remains a *hot* topic, even though it's been unseasonably cold. I believe without *global warming* I'd have frozen to death last winter. Some might feel sorry for our erstwhile senator/politician turned scientist because it's hard to argue a position that is contrary to what people observe. St. Augustine in the 5th century stated that even the Church should never hold a position that is contrary to observable fact.

And this is the crux of the matter; science is not religion, and climate change issues have become more religion than science. Science is based on observable reality, not faith. Unfortunately, our trust in climate science has been shaken with the scandal of *Climategate*. As you recall, the principle climate "scientists" of the United Nations at the University of East Anglia were caught fudging data, limiting contrary viewpoints and lying to everyone, perhaps even Al-gore.

My brother Tom is a geologist and is the most knowledgeable science-based person I know regarding climate science. His article about a year ago in the *Knox Focus* was the standard for a non-expert like me. Tom is a skeptic of man-made global warming, and I have to admit I don't trust the UN, its scientists at the IPCC and I don't trust Al-gore, the politician-activist-entrepreneur whose home in Nashville uses more electricity than twelve average Nashville homes. And I don't want to discuss Al's private jet and his new home in Santa Barbara, whose entrance is below the flood line (if his predictions of rising sea levels are correct). The real casualties of all this hype are the taxpayers, the discipline of science and the graduates of my alma mater, the University of Tennessee.

I hate donning the mantle of victim-hood, but the Al-gorian climate religion has branded me a skeptic and the UT diplomas my wife and I earned through years of hard work have been lessened by Al-gore's *doctorate*. You may argue that his honorary degree doesn't directly affect mine, but I disagree. It certainly lessens the other honorary UT doctorates given to Dolly Parton and Howard Baker for their lifetimes of service to the people of Tennessee.

What I really object to is the politicization of academics and science by Al-gore and his ilk. It makes my job of caring for and advising patients on the basis of scientific data all the more difficult. Why should anyone believe science when "researchers" fudge their results to maintain their grants?

You may have noticed that virtually all our institutions are under assault. A few examples are Christianity and even the American way. How do we know what is right or what we should do? Once we might have asked our minister or our doctor; but these are now in doubt just like the news media. The ancients would have studied history to discover a course of action, but not post-modern man.

One of the tenets of our post-modern era is that there is no absolute. This can take the form of relativism, where a community standard or a nation determines what is right. Extending that logic, any other culture might consider their standards as equally just or virtuous. Subjectivism holds that each of us determines our own sense of morality. It gets pretty crazy if there isn't some semblance of a standard, a touchstone. The ancients referred to a standard as the *tertium quid* or a Rosetta stone that serves as the standard measuring stick of life.

I was once lost in an existentialist standard-less free fall. I learned to accept the Way and embrace the mysteries of life. I am still a scientist, an empiricist, a Doubting Thomas who says "show me the data." Unfortunately, Al-gore has fallen far short of that standard and UT has let me down. So I'll just keep looking **Up** for the answers.

We live at the bottom of a sea of air. Our astronauts can actually see the atmosphere that surrounds the Earth. But when we breathe in or look out we don't see anything even though it's there. You will certainly notice the absence of air if you go high enough in an airplane or if you go to the top of Mt. Everest. In these rarefied places no matter how hard you breathe there is not enough air/oxygen to sustain life without artificial airline cabin pressurization or oxygen supplements. I can even feel the effects of thinner air as I huff and puff up the stairs at my brother and sister-in-law's house in the Colorado Mountains that is 8000 feet above sea level.

Have you ever watched a fish when taken out of the water? It's not a pretty sight and I find myself empathizing with the poor creature. I've had the "air knocked out of me" a few times and perhaps this is what the fish feels as it gasps for air. A fish's gills are designed to remove oxygen from water and are useless in our thin air. However, human lungs are very efficient at removing the oxygen we need from the atmosphere; at least as long as our lungs are healthy and we're not at a really high altitude.

As we leave sea level, air pressure begins to fall and as a result it is increasingly difficult to extract enough oxygen from the thinning air. But, this is rarely an issue at low altitudes and commercial airlines provide pressurization equivalent to about 8000 feet elevation. However, this level of air pressure may be insufficient for a patient with severe lung disease and it may be necessary for your doctor to arrange for oxygen supplements for air travel.

Try to visualize your lungs as a bunch of grapes. The stalk is analogous to the windpipe and the ever smaller stems are like the smaller airways of the bronchial tree which end in millions of alveoli (air sacks) like grapes at the ends of stems. These tiny alveolar *balloons,* if spread out, would have the collective surface area of a tennis court and function as oxygen and carbon dioxide exchangers. As we breathe in, air and oxygen move down the air ducts and finally into air sacks. Oxygen moves through the alveolar walls and is absorbed into the blood stream. Also, carbon dioxide waste moves from the blood stream into the air sacks and is then breathed out as we exhale. (I wonder what each of our *carbon offsets* will be in Obama's Cap and Trade legislation since we all produce carbon dioxide)

Surprisingly, shortness of breath with lung disease results when you can't breathe out and empty your lungs, rather than difficulty inhaling. It might feel like your big brother sitting on your chest squeezing the breath out of you, but actually the lungs can't empty and become overinflated in asthma attacks and in the damaged lungs of COPD (Chronic Obstructive Lung Disease). Your lungs become like overinflated balloons making it impossible to take a deep breath.

One of my all time favorite books is **Pilgrim at Tinker Creek** by Annie Dillard. It was her first book and she won a Pulitzer Prize for this jewel of a novel. Among her many stories and observations is a description of the plant protein *chlorophyll* and its similarity to the human protein *hemoglobin*. Chlorophyll exists as a one hundred and thirty-six atom ring structure with magnesium at the center. If you substitute iron for the magnesium at the center of the ring structure you get hemoglobin.

Hemoglobin carries oxygen in our blood stream. Plants produce the oxygen we need, and the carbon (as carbon dioxide) we breathe out is used by plants, driven by the photosynthesis of chlorophyll to grow the plant.

What an amazing symbiosis! We are a part of the whole that some have seen as an example of *Gaia*.

Food for thought…

Much of my day is spent separating the wheat from the chaff. Patients tell me their stories, I examine them and I decide whether their concerns are serious or just aggravations. Fortunately, serious problems are less common than the proverbial bumps along the *aches* of life. However, a good clinician pays attention because seemingly minor concerns can be the tip of a medical iceberg.

Atrial fibrillation is a common heart problem. This arrhythmia of the heart often causes palpitations or weakness, as it did in the man I admitted into the hospital the other night. At other times the condition may be relatively silent until a disastrous stroke occurs. So what is heart disorder and what do you do about it?

I'm a big believer in eye contact and touching. The latter may sound a bit strange in our politically correct world, but numerous studies have shown that patients perceive a doctor as caring when he not only listens, but makes eye and physical contact during medical evaluations. I make it a point to listen to everyone's heart and lungs when they visit me for care. And sometimes when I listen the heart rhythm is fast and irregular, and reflective of atrial fibrillation.

We are born with a pacemaker that resides in an upper chamber of the heart. This natural pacemaker coordinates the heart rate and rhythm. Unfortunately, this pacemaker ages along with the rest of the body, and can be affected by other heart diseases or thyroid dysfunction.

If the heart *jumps out of rhythm* an EKG (electrocardiogram) is used to confirm the diagnosis, and simple blood tests and a chest X-ray are used to check for other problems, especially thyroid over-activity.

A logical goal is to put the heart back into its normal rhythm and to control the often rapid heart rate. The heart is not designed to function with a sustained rapid heart rate just as your car's idle isn't supposed to race the engine. Atrial fibrillation also causes a loss of pumping efficiency of the heart and can cause angina or heart failure.

The immediate treatment of atrial fibrillation is medications to slow the abnormal heart rate, and sometimes these medications can restore heart's normal rhythm. One might think that restoring the heart rhythm to normal would be the best treatment. A large clinical trial was designed to test whether it's better to simply control the fast heart rhythm or use other measures to put the heart back into rhythm such as *cardioversion* (shocking the heart back into rhythm). It turns out that both therapy options are equally appropriate. If rhythm control is chosen, the patient has to take lifelong medications to prevent recurrent atrial fibrillation. And if the heart rate option is chosen lifelong medication to prevent blood clots are often necessary.

Most of us are familiar with the Tennessee River from boating or walking along its shores. We've all seen debris and flotsam on the river, especially after a storm. Sometimes the debris gets trapped in back waters where the flow is sluggish. Unfortunately, atrial fibrillation causes stagnant flow that can produce clots which may break free and cause a disastrous stroke.

To prevent blood clots doctors give anticoagulants such as warfarin. These *anti-clotting* drugs counteract the heightened clotting tendency in the dysfunctional heart. It's tricky business to use these medications which produce a hemophiliac tendency. A measure of the right dose is the so-called "PT" test that is now referred to as the INR or PT-INR test. The goal is to maintain the number between two and three for most problems. This requires frequent blood tests and adjustments of the dose because either too much medication leads to bleeding or too little may allow a clot to form and a stroke to occur.

Perhaps this is more than you cared to know about atrial fibrillation, but then maybe it touches your heart!

The world is changing right in front of my eyes. I realize that I'm more resistant to change than I once was, but perhaps that's in part because I've learned what works through the school of hard knocks.

Doctors, like everyone else, begin to think about retirement when their priorities change or when they sense that it's harder to keep up with the demands of medical practice. Recently, an ER (emergency room) colleague of mine shook his head as he watched me admit the seventh patient in six hours to the hospital. "Ferguson," he said, "I'll tell the next person who wonders if you're getting too old that you can still work harder than most." But, I have to admit that it's tougher than it used to be and harder to keep up with the latest in medicine. Though I still regularly read seven medical journals, I find that I've become more interested in history, philosophy and religion. And I find that writing has become my passion. Writing will never be my vocation, but it has become my **avocation**. Creative writing gives me joy and is an outlet for teaching beyond the patient in front of me.

A friend of mine likes to say that, "You're either growing or you're dying." That's probably a good philosophical perspective. A fundamental principle of the universe is entropy – energy systems, like a top or a clock, wind down. You have to resist this basic principle of physics by exercising your body and your mind. That's why I still push myself; I want to keep growing; I'm not ready to retire or die!

I've often mentioned the electronic prescribing system in my medical practice. I'm not a techy person, but I love my iPhone. In fact, I'm so enthusiastic about my ability to access definitions and the compendium of human knowledge that I'm at work incorporating this technological concept into my second novel. But, there's a downside to these contrivances. I was listening to a patient's heart yesterday and all at once his cell phone in his shirt pocket rang and made my teeth rattle through the stethoscope's amplified sound. I believe in the personal touch and always make a point of listening to the heart and lungs of virtually every patient I see. I've just got to be more careful in the future or I'll be deaf!

Words are the tools we use to express ourselves – another *Ferg-ism*. Think about it; if you have no words-tools you'll never be able to tell your story. I'm a collector of stories and verbal tools. Some of you have questioned why I sprinkle an essay with a word that might not be in everyone's **lexicon**. I would challenge you to ask Mr. Google or a dictionary about the words you don't know as this will foster growth in the tool shed of your mind.

I have to admit that I was stumped recently when a patient called me and mumbled, "Doc! I'm avomikin!" Neither my iPhone nor the Net would have helped me as I struggled to listen to the **vernacular** amidst the rest of his story. It turns out he was sick and vomiting! Remember, words are tools, so use good ones with careful **elocution**.

Sometimes it's necessary to learn street synonyms for Mr. Webster's words. When I was in training at an inner city hospital I learned that patients understood anemia as *low- blood* and hypertension as *high-blood*. Syphilis was a scourge in the ghetto and was known as *bad blood*. Sickle cell anemia is a terrible disease associated with anemia and recurrent bouts of severe pain. You can understand why it was known as *sick-as-hell anemia*. When I returned to Knoxville to practice internal medicine I learned that words and phrases had regional **nuances** here as well. A *bealed-ear* represented an ear ache and a *rizen on the pajama* referred to a boil on a…uh… sensitive area below the naval. Recently my patient said, "Doc, my nature's gone." I'll leave you to contemplate what he was trying to tell me.

Someone once said that life is an education. This comes from John Dewey who said, "Education is not a preparation for life, but is life itself." The ancient Greeks had a word for a consuming curiosity and quest for knowledge. They called it *gnosis*.

I've still got a passion for life and learning. I've still got my edge. In fact, my routine of daily journaling (as a form of devotion) and the *Knox Focus* have given me a new lease on life. I'm blessed, and I continue to grow!

You'd have to be in a coma to be unaware of the crisis in Washington and our nation. We are broke, and yet the President and the Democrats refuse serious spending cuts and ask for another extension on the National credit card which is maxed out. The "experts" tell us to trust Washington because they know better than John Q Public; we at least understand that you can't continue to spend more than you have. Both parties and presidents for decades have done this, but now it's crunch time. We either say, "No more!" and begin to turn the country around or it's all over. The President says we have to "Eat our peas," but soon there will be no peas to eat.

I really hate wasting column space on the budget crisis, but this is a crisis, rather than the manufactured ones that the media trots out on a regular basis to foment angst. Remember, the journalistic mantra is "If it bleeds, it leads." In other words, you can sell more newspapers and advertising space on television with a weather crisis or sensational murders. Wouldn't it be nice to wake some morning and not worry about whether the mullah's in Iran have acquired the bomb? Wouldn't it be nice to be assured that your life's work and savings, and your children's future, were not in danger of destruction by Congress and the President? Unfortunately, we have ignored our spending sickness for years and have entrusted our future to Washington. How's that working for you? *We The People* now recognize the crisis, but it may be too late. Even now, Obama, Reid, Boehner and the boys want to again kick the can (debt problem) down the road, to use the current euphemism.

Do you realize that there is an automatic increase to the Federal budget every year predicated on projected needs and growth? Folks, there isn't any growth and even if we cut the budget a fraction there remains a built-in increase! I've come to the conclusion that we have two choices: increase the debt *limit* again with the politician's token spending cuts, and accept the end of our economy and country; **or** stop this national suicide by cutting spending to levels of 2008 while paying interest on our debts to prevent default. These measures should continue until our house is put in order. The first choice is certain destruction; the second choice gives us a chance to recover.

I have called my Congressman and Senators and again urged them to stand on principle. I urged them to adopt the President's bipartisan Debt Commission recommendations published in December 2010. Unfortunately, President Obama tossed out Simpson and Bowle's recommendations, while at the same time the Democratic Congress and Senate in December again refused to pass a budget. I suspect my exhortations will go unheeded or be too little too late.

But enough of this gloom and doom! The Teacher in Ecclesiastes taught us that we should enjoy life, food, wine, and love our spouses. He said we should do our jobs to the best of our abilities, respect the Lord and keep His commandments. And we must seek a relationship with Him. This advice rendered 3000 years ago by purportedly the smartest man in history (Solomon) gives meaning to my life and is far better than the incessant bickering over government policy.

Two weeks ago another writer in The Focus described a hilarious mouse story and reminded me how important humor is. We need some levity to lighten our load. Sometimes you've just got to laugh, so I'll close with a story that might give you a chuckle.

One cold wintery night while I was all "snug in my bed," my wife Becky squeezed my arm and anxiously whispered, "Someone's in our bedroom!" As I struggled to clear my sleepy head and sit up, she hissed, "Be still and listen!" It was pitch black as I struggled to listen. What I heard, as I waited for Norman Bates to stab us to death, was a rustling across the room that seemed to move along the baseboard. I considered my options of waiting to be clubbed or confronting the intruder. Finally, I steeled myself to turn on the light and reach for my revolver in the bedside drawer. It was then that I saw the flying squirrel.

Flying squirrels are creepy looking things with eyes disproportionate to their tiny bodies because they are nocturnal. Actually, the poor thing was in my bedroom seeking shelter on a miserably cold winter night. Becky and I decided not to swat the creature, but to try and usher it to the front door and sweep it outside where it belonged.

To the tiny squirrel I'm sure we appeared as terrifying giants with our brooms and our robes and *little else*. We finally maneuvered the squirrel to the door which Becky was to open so that I could usher our guest back into nature. What we didn't count on was the cat at the door. As the door swung open the cat saw the squirrel and pounced. The last thing I saw was that creepy-looking thing disappearing up my leg, beneath my robe, towards my "*junk*." Folks, who says white men can't jump?!

It's hard to be objective about yourself. This is why doctors and patients are advised to seek medical help rather than treat themselves. However, let's be honest: we all prescribe for ourselves for minor issues.

If my memory serves me correctly, I once wrote a story about the scientific method and how doctors think. The ancient Greeks were the first to apply observational reality. Instead of imagining the world around them as caused by magic or the intervention of gods, they applied careful observation and then used logic to discover how things work.

These days we are bombarded with information. Just recently a patient asked me about the latest diet advised by Dr. Oz. Another asked me if cinnamon would really cure his diabetes as suggested by a commercial. And as I drove home to write this essay, an infomercial recommended "Dr. Block's Super Food," which is said to contain "50 different organic vegetables and fruits" all in a condensed capsule formulation which will restore vigor and promote weight loss. This particular product did not purport to improve a man's virility as do so many others.

I was sharing my own aches and pains recently with a patient and he recommended Mega Red joint care. He **averred** that it had really helped his joint pain. I told him that I was glad his knee pain was better, but the scientist in me was skeptical. I thought it was more likely his diet and weight loss had helped his knee pain.

It must have been a weak moment or the rainy day that was making my knee pain worse, because I found myself in the nutraceutical section of my local drugstore. I was there to pick up a prescription, but as I waited I decided to look up the ingredients of Mega Red. Aside from the "proprietary ingredients," the formulation contained krill oil and hyaluronic acid, a constituent of cartilage.

Cartilage is present in the lobes of our ears and the knee joints. It is smooth and spongy absorbing the shock of walking. Osteoarthritis is primarily a disease of cartilage so you can see why an agent able to repair damaged cartilage would be desirable. About a decade ago a flurry of medical papers extolled the virtues of chondroitin sulfate and glucosamine as able to repair damaged cartilage. However, later clinical studies cast doubts on the earlier findings.

Hyaluronic acid, chondroitin and glucosamine are all building blocks of the cartilage that covers the endplates of bones. Cartilage is naturally smooth, and most of us have observed the smooth aspect of the head of a soup bone. The damaged cartilage surface in degenerative arthritis is analogous to a pockmarked driveway. The hypothesis was that by ingesting the building blocks of cartilage the damaged surface could be repaired like resurfacing an old road. However, resurfacing cannot repair potholes!

It never made sense to me how you could swallow a pill of chondroitin/glucosamine or hyaluronic acid and have these substances find their way to a diseased knee. Nonetheless, early studies showed that those people taking significant doses of these formulations had less joint pain. It is interesting that similar proteins obtained from a rooster's comb and then injected into an arthritic joint improves pain, though recent studies have cast doubt on the effectiveness of these joint injections as well.

These thoughts flashed through my mind as I studied the Mega Red formulation. I decided to run my own pseudo-scientific experiment using Becky and me as guinea pigs. Medical science works best with the results of prospective, randomized, double blinded, placebo-controlled medical studies. In this type of study design neither the patient nor the doctor knows who is taking the study drug or a placebo that is determined by random assignment.

The best I could manage was to quantitate our knee discomfort and then use Mega Red for four weeks before reevaluating the pain in our knees. We also planned a follow-up two-week trial without the nutraceutical. I've recommended this same "internal" study design for patients who want to try chondroitin/glucosamine. I would add one caveat to this protocol: count your pills when you come home from the drug store. We think Mega Red shorted us!

You may have heard of the recent sensational study from Northwestern University regarding regular or casual use of marijuana. The research study which appears in the Journal of Neuroscience showed that daily marijuana use or even twice a month usage was associated with impairment of "working memory." This study used a sophisticated MRI brain scanning technique and also showed that two areas in the brain associated with "emotions, making decisions, and motivation" were structurally abnormal in those who use marijuana. And heavier usage of marijuana was associated with even greater abnormalities.

For me it is troubling that two states have legalized recreational use of marijuana. There is some scientific evidence for medicinal use of marijuana in association with cancer and possibly chronic pain syndromes. There are no studies that show the safety of recreational use and it seems premature for our country to legalize this otherwise controlled substance.

Personally, I find it objectionable to think of deeply inhaling any partially combusted (burned) plant fiber, since we know that inhaling tobacco smoke (another partially combusted plant leaf) is carcinogenic. And now science raises the specter that the use of marijuana causes structural abnormalities of the brain as well as memory problems and the so-called amotivation syndrome.

A lot is said these days about athletes being role models. Given these new scientific findings, should our President (who was a heavy user of marijuana) and Eric Holder (head of the Justice Department) be supporting legalization of marijuana?

John Adams, another president of the United States, once said, "Facts are such troublesome things." Are you listening, Mr. President?

I once wrote an essay maintaining that dogs smile. Furthermore, many people, including my nurse LuAnn, say that dogs and animals have souls. More on that in a minute, but as proof of a soulful smile, I offer the non photo-shopped picture of "Captain Jack" helping me (JD) pilot a front loader. Gentlemen and ladies of the jury, I rest my case. Surely this is evidence of a grin from ear to ear.

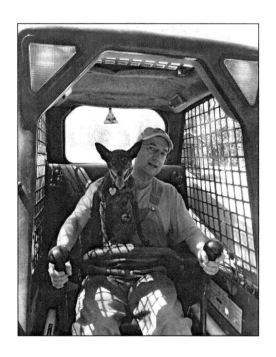

My readers must know by now that human behavior intrigues me. We are said to be made in the image of The Creator and endowed with reason which most of the time tempers our passions. In the Wisdom writings the Psalmist said that we are "fearfully and wonderfully made." I offer as evidence the smile of a baby. It's even more magical than a puppy!

I've become a student of my grandson's smiles. Oakley smiles and laughs out loud now; in fact, his first recorded laugh was in response to and what has become known in our family as JD's dance. JD is short for Jim-Dad a name that works for both of my grandsons. Oakley also entertains us with squeals of delight, but can let you know of his displeasure when his attendants are slow to produce the desired bottle. However, I'm more intrigued by his evolving repertoire of facial expressions that I see as nuanced forms of communication without words.

"Where did he learn that bashful look?" Becky asked me one day. I had no answer, but it made me consider how we learn to smile and what a smile's purpose is.

I've read that it takes many more muscles to frown than it does to smile. I wonder why a smile connotes friendliness where a frown or a scowl does not. Why do we see a smile as esthetically pleasing? I heard once that a newborn monkey, when placed in a cage with a snake, will go berserk. Surely, the tiny monkey didn't learn this survival attitude from its mother, but perhaps it did. Maybe the answer lies in genetic memory where certain survival skills are imparted to newborns at conception, when the full complement of DNA is present to produce a monkey, a Captain Jack, or a human baby that can suckle and smile.

Perhaps Oakley has genetic recognition that our smiles can be trusted and come from love. However, I believe he's learning to nuance his feelings beyond hunger and pleasure with the more advanced facial expressions of communication. He probably learns from us as we contort our faces to make him giggle, a sound that is more melodious and cherished than Mozart's clarinet concerto. Oakley doesn't *speak* yet, but he communicates plenty.

I've got a new book of anatomy that should be much more patient-friendly than the one I used in medical school in 1973. Experts say that there are at least six hundred and forty muscles in the human body and about 40 of these are in the face. It is the contraction of these facial muscles that move our jaw (mandible) and stretch the skin of our face to produce facial expressions. I'm not sure the anatomist included the muscles of a protruded tongue in his tally of expressive facial musculature.

In my Triad Group we're reading a deep philosophical book by Soren Kierkegaard, which I can't recommend to anyone. However, the author raises interesting questions about a person's spirit, or the sense of self, that got me to thinking beyond just the conscious awareness of myself and others. Indisputably, we all have a body and a sense of self. But, so does my dog Jack. Some might argue that the sense of self resides in that ill-defined area we call the soul. If that is true, then animals and Jack have souls. That intriguing perspective once drove me to consider a vegetarian lifestyle. It didn't last because I abhor tofu and I came to the conclusion that I was designed as an omnivore. It's hard to override design specifications.

What is the conscience and where does it reside? Is the conscience what defines the sense of self or one's soul? The ancients held that the life force was associated with the lungs and the breath of life. Later, the heart was recognized as the primal force because when it stopped beating consciousness and conscience ceased. We moderns think that the sense of self, our conscience, and perhaps the soul is incorporated within our very complicated nervous system that extends throughout our entire body. In a sense, our neural net defines our body and mind!

Like the U-Tube video, *The Honey Badger*, Jack doesn't care much about the philosophical musings of his front-loader co-captain. Though he is a noble creation, he thinks less deeply than his master and therefore he doesn't see as far or reach for the stars like his master.

Someone once imagined that the first prayer uttered by a human was long ago when our proverbial ancestor looked up at the stars one a dark night and said, "Ahhh."

What a soulful/Spirit-filled moment. I'll bet our ancestor was smiling, and I'll bet the Creator was smiling back!

The Crèche - December 21, 2011

Every year I wait in anticipation for the Christmas Spirit, and it always comes, eventually. In years past I've mentioned that Becky and I love Christmas movies and we watch all of them before the Holidays are over. This year for some reason we started with *Scrooged* starring Bill Murray. It's a story about a cynical man finding the Christmas Spirit. I'm not as pessimistic as Murray's character, but I have to admit it's been a tough year and I'm *hoping for change.*

Last Saturday my daughter Jenny, son-in-law Ryand, grandson Noah and my brother Tom accompanied Becky and me to our neighbor's tree farm in Townsend. We went en masse to cut The Ferguson Family's Christmas Tree as in the movie *Christmas Vacation.* Ryand and I get along well because our favorite movie depicts the Griswold family with "kith and kin" at Christmas. However, we didn't forget our chainsaw like Clark Griswold, and I didn't get a tree that was too big this year, thanks to Becky's restraint. I even got the tree up and the lights on before JP's graduation party.

In past essays I've spoken of our refugee friends from Burundi and their son JP who has just earned his high school diploma. The party was to honor his achievement and everyone came. They even helped add ornaments to our tree. Unfortunately, JP's parents, Joseph and his wife Maria, are often on the outside in gatherings because of the language barrier between English and their native tongue Kirundi.

As I watched JP open gifts and cards I thought about how little we know about his Mom and Dad. Translation is difficult and imperfect at best. I understand this because of my medical mission work in Guatemala where we often had to translate English to Spanish and then Spanish to Quiché, the local Mayan dialect, and then back again. But as I thought about Joseph and Maria on the periphery of the party, I realized that I do know them because I know their son, JP and their other children.

Becky loves the Joseph family and a deal. In fact, I've told her that I'm going to put on her gravestone that "She never paid retail." I've observed that women shop and men buy. If I find what I want, I buy it. If Becky finds what she wants even with a good price, she keeps looking until she's convinced she's found a deal. I don't complain much because she's an exceptional woman and manager of our home.

Years ago Becky found a beautiful crèche (manger scene) at the old downtown Watson's Department store. She couldn't believe the low price which seemed incongruous with the obvious quality of the Christian icon. (Incidentally, Saint

Francis of Assisi is credited with creating the manger scene in the 1200s.) It was not until she got home that she realized the bargain resulted from the absence of Jesus' father Joseph in the assembled crèche.

We have two visions of the Christmas story from the Gospels of Matthew and Luke which tend to become blended in our modern minds. One Gospel describes the lineage of Jesus through his mother, Mary (Maria), and the other emphasizes Jesus' father, Joseph. Mary is mentioned many other times in The Greatest Story Ever Told, but Joseph, the father, fades from history after the first few chapters of Matthew's and Luke's stories. What happened to Joseph? Did he die? Was he only there to lend his name to Jesus or to play a bit part?

Becky has done community theatre for years and in her role as Grace in *The Best Christmas Pageant Ever,* her character opines that "There are no small parts, only small actors." Well, Jesus' father, Joseph could not have been a small actor. We may not know much about him because the Bible is less a book of facts than it is a book of truth which is only realized in the hearts and minds of each of us. However, I believe we do know Joseph because we know Jesus. We are told that Jesus "grew in wisdom and stature and in favor with God and men." I'm convinced that Jesus' success as a human being was molded by his father as well as his mother.

We hear a lot these days about single parents, non-traditional couples, broken homes and marriage versus civil unions. I believe the most important job you will ever have is raising your child. Excluding abusive and dangerous situations, I believe it is imperative that children receive the wisdom of male and female parents, and that both should focus on what is best for their child rather than what the parent needs.

Jesus once said that if you "know me you know The Father." Yes, that is truth. And I know our Maria and Joseph because I know their son JP.
Merry Christmas to all of my readers, and thanks for following my stories in our **Knoxville Focus.**

I ended last week's essay with observations of Rafe Hollister, moonshiner and *philosopher* on the **Andy Griffith Show**. I open this week's missive with another observation of Rafe. People often greet each other with the euphemistic question, "How are you?" but without the expectation of a serious answer. Actually, we often already know how people are doing from their body language which speaks loudly to those with observational skills. I think I'll adopt Rafe's response when people ask me how I'm doing. "Midl'n, just midl'n," says it all for me these days. Lately, I'm just *hang'n* in there.

I recently read a survey that recorded a serious level of dissatisfaction within the Millennial Generation. This oft quoted survey described Millennials as frustrated that they will not be as successful as their parents, the Baby Boomers. It is well known that the Baby Boomers reaped the benefits of unparalleled freedom and opportunity that came from the sacrifices of the Greatest Generation. A patient of that era recently told me that when she was growing up "Chicken was a Sunday-only meal." Now it's available for breakfast, lunch and supper seven days a week.

Perhaps the dissatisfaction of Millennials is a result of the rotten economy and job scarcity despite the unprecedented level of education in our graduates. Perhaps it's the realization that nine million American jobs are gone forever and that three fourths of new jobs are only part-time. Perhaps the notion of American exceptionalism has been pilloried in the halls of academia for so long that young people have lost confidence in themselves and their country, and now expect someone to give them a great job with benefits and lots of free time. Our medical group used a renowned national agency to find a new physician for the group who would embrace a traditional office medical practice and care for their patients when hospitalized. We couldn't find anyone and so my partners became my former partners and left hospital practice altogether.

Ennui is a word that comes to us from French. It means a lack of enthusiasm or a sense of weariness. This mood pervades our country now and is as palpable as a swollen knee. There are exceptions, but more and more I sense frustration or an "I don't care attitude," even among physicians. A sense of resignation is in our hospital, in my patients and in me, where often the best I can muster these days is "Midl'n, just midl'n."

There is a verse in the 2nd epistle of Timothy that I love and identify with. (I know you're not supposed to end a sentence in a preposition, but sometimes avoiding this grammatical rule makes prose seem excessively formal and stiff, so I'll apologize to grammarians and my editor-wife and proceed.) Late in Paul's career and life the Apostle and philosopher would say, "I fought the good fight,

169

I finished the race and kept the faith." These days I'm trying to do so myself as medicine becomes increasingly a job to so many, instead of a life calling or profession.

My patient awakened in the middle of the night with the sensation that his face felt funny. As he rushed to the bathroom and a mirror he noticed that his right arm was weak and clumsy as well. His drooping face was confirmed by his alarmed wife, so they rushed to the nearest emergency room where a stroke was diagnosed by the ER (emergency room) doctor and a CAT scan.

As my patient was awaiting admission to the hospital for more tests, the emergency physician told him that a neurologist was coming to see him for a neurological consultation. Imagine my surprise when my patient and his wife later described the robot who came to see him escorted by the ER nurse. You see, the neurologist was in Atlanta and the consultation was done by Skype! Apparently, there aren't enough neurologists in Knoxville to see stroke patients at night. I shouldn't be surprised because years ago I learned that emergency CT scans in the middle of the night are often interpreted by radiologists in Australia who are awake at 2 am EST.

Bob Dylan once crooned, "Oh, the times they are a chang'n." I agree, and the times demand changes. You've heard the advice that we should choose to be glad **in** our circumstances, but not necessarily **for** the troubles before us. As I age I sometimes say thank you that I'm still around to even have circumstances. I've asked many people if they would like to be sixteen again. However, there's a catch: you don't get to take the lessons of life with you. In my nonscientific survey all have chosen wisdom and wrinkles over youth and its confusion.

My hospitalized patient with pneumonia was a study in the conservation of energy and reminded me of a beach ball. As I entered her room I looked for her high energy husband, and after examining her I asked how his recent retirement was going for both of them. She said, "It's like living with a squirrel, Dr. Ferguson!" I managed a sympathetic smile while secretly wishing that this overweight lady had some of his energy and activity. I quipped, "You know it takes time to break in new shoes, and you don't throw old shoes away unless they're worn out." She got the message and got well, and went home to her slightly *nutty* partner.

My life partner and wife tolerates my increasingly frequent midl'n attitudes and encourages me. It is said that a physician should heal himself. Maybe he should listen to both his spiritual mentor and his wife. After all the choice of a good attitude is the best medicine.

Have you ever gone to the refrigerator and found something unidentifiable in a Tupperware container? There's a great line by Walter Matthau in the *Odd Couple* movie. His character Oscar is hosting a poker party and announces to his buddies, "I've got green sandwiches and brown sandwiches – it's either very new cheese or very old meat." As I recall there wasn't a high demand for these unidentifiable edibles. None of us would put something in our mouths if we didn't know what it was – except perhaps Ratatouille's brother, and he's a Disney cartoon rat!

Honestly, it amazes me how many patients have no clue what medications they're taking. Some entrust their pills to their spouse, and sometimes this is understandable if they're confused, can't read or too infirm to administer a complicated therapy program. And I understand that medications are often confusing to patients; but folks you must take some responsibility for what you put in your mouth.

Last week I was trained to use a new computer-based medication reconciliation program at our hospital. All the doctors who still take care of hospitalized patients are taking this training which involves patients/families, nurses/pharmacists and doctors. It often takes a team effort to figure out what patients are taking when they enter the hospital. Sick patients and distraught families often have trouble giving an accurate list of medications or how the medications are being used.

In general, I think Americans take too many pills. Part of the problem is that many think the answer to their problems reside in a pill. As an example, people frequently ask me about diet pills. I've been in medicine forty years and the hope of an effective and safe diet pill remains elusive. Sometimes I tell patients that I was once fat and teased mercilessly as a kid. I made up my mind in middle school that my will was stronger than my stomach's growls. I vowed never to be fat again and I still watch my "diet" to this day.

Perhaps our pill problems are analogous to those of Congress who continues to make laws and never cancel the obsolete ones. We doctors often just add to a patient's cocktail as each new problem arises. Late one night I admitted another doctor's patient to the hospital and that patient still holds the "world" record medication list. How could that poor lady take thirsty-six different medications every day? I didn't think it was possible, and if by chance she was able to choke down all those pills I wondered what all that medicine would do to a person.
When I see a patient in the office my nurse and I go over the medication list separately. It's amazing that after two careful surveys I've discovered that the list is still inaccurate 25% of the time. People don't consider vitamins, herbs and supplements as medication. And patients often use non-prescription drugs like Tylenol, Aleve or Motrin without considering their interaction with prescription

medications such as warfarin or Plavix. The French have a saying that you are what you eat. I believe it's true with medications as well.

I'm always looking to eliminate or combine medications in a simpler way to improve compliance with vital medications. I once had an elderly lady who was always after me to reduce her pill list. When I could do no more she gruffly huffed and said, "Humph; you're a city boy aren't you?"

I thought, oh no, she's going to unload on me. I thought quickly and managed to reply, "Well, yes, Ma'am, I am." And that's when the lesson began.

She said, "Have you ever watched a chicken eat?" Puzzled, but curious where this was going, I told her yes I've seen chickens plucking in a barnyard. She then said, "Well, at breakfast every morning, I pore out your pills onto the table, and with a glass of water in my hand I pluck up those pills like corn in the barnyard." I carry that vision in my mind almost thirty years later.

Many have observed that teenagers consider themselves immortal, bullet proof and perhaps invisible. Of course this is tongue-in-cheek, but it reflects an attitude that nothing will happen to them. As we get older we realize there are consequences for our choices, but apparently the child in us remains because we believe that the system or the government will take care of us and we needn't worry. Folks, that is magical thinking and dangerous. As hard as I try it isn't enough; you must help me know what pills you are putting into your mouth. The Cheshire Cat once said, "If you don't know where you're going, any road'll do." That doesn't work with medication.

Maybe Americans in the 21st century just want to be taken care of instead of exercising individual responsibility and freedom. However, I can tell you that the medical system, no matter how sophisticated, cannot replace your personal responsibility or your family's participation in your care. Furthermore, I can assure you with the certainty of forty years of experience, that things are even more complicated now, and care is increasingly problematic in the New Order.

Be responsible and help your doctor help you!

In January I will have been in medicine forty years. This comprises two-thirds of my life and virtually all of my adult life. I went to medical school in January 1973. The world is dramatically different now than it was then. There were no CAT scans 'til I was in my internal medicine residency. Only Star Trek's Dr. McCoy had the equivalent of an MRI in his hand-held tricorder. Automated blood chemistry profiles were just becoming available in the mid-1970s, and we certainly didn't have the advanced technology diabetics take for granted to check their blood sugar at home.

In those days we were trained as men of science and would never have mentioned our faith, even if we had any. I'll admit there was a time when I thought science was a god. The ancient Greeks would have considered this the height of hubris, and knowing what I know now, I would agree. I had a lot of facts in my noggin through those early years. Some of these I organized into a compendium of working knowledge. I'm wiser now because I've learned to use this education and experience prudently.

I felt "free at last" when beepers became available, and I could move about when on-call, even if I had to plug dimes into pay phones along the roadside. Yes, I said dimes, which later became quarters. Now you'd have trouble finding a pay phone. Have you ever wondered why doctors are no longer paged to call the Doctor's Exchange at UT football games? Now, we've exchanged our beepers for computers in our pockets (smart phones) which connect us to the vast database of the internet. As the Russian comedian Smirnoff once said, "What a country!"

The doctors of my era were trained in the philosophy of the Hippocratic Oath. Hippocrates was an ancient Greek physician and promulgated a professional code of ethics for doctors. There is much in the Oath that is no longer germane to our post-modern era, but his insistence that physicians work for the betterment of each **individual** patient is fundamental in my training. How interesting that Obama's bioethical advisor is Ezekiel Emanuel – Rahm Emanuel's brother – who says that doctors should no longer be trained in the Hippocratic philosophy. Doctor Emanuel says we should be more attentive to **societal** needs than the patient before us.

When I first went into practice I emulated the senior physicians on the medical staff at University Hospital. Their motto was, "We practice what we teach." They taught me, I taught medical students and residents, and we taught each other, nurses and patients. Professionalism was the raison d'être of those days rather than the industry of medicine and the business model which drives medical care these days.

173

A cross country plane trip is a good metaphor for my life and career in medicine. During the first third of the journey I prepared myself by tanking up on experiences and education which enabled me to race down the runway and take off into the future. My wife Becky and I together soared into the proverbial stratosphere and achieved cruising altitude as we built a family supported by my medical practice. During any plane trip there comes a time when the pilot powers down and begins his descent toward his final destination. I tell myself that I'm not on the final approach nor have I lowered my landing gear. Something tells me that the journey is not over and it's not time for a landing and a taxi to the hanger of retirement. But it's closer than it was.

There seem to be fewer doctors in the hospital these days. I'm a dinosaur; I'm one of the few internists who still make rounds and care for my patients in the hospital. When I was president of Summit Medical Group we established the hospitalist system known in Knoxville as STAT CARE. It is these hospital doctors who now care for patients whose doctors no longer go to the hospital. Our hospitalists do a fine job, but I persist in the belief that my patients chose me as their doctor, and I have a responsibility to be there for them in their hour of greatest need, especially when things are scary, confusing and they are most vulnerable. Maybe, this is another old fashioned concept that needs to be replaced by the "new reality."

One of my aphorisms says that "there is always someone stronger, smarter or prettier than you are." As an internist and geriatrician I'm glad to have the expertise of those more specialized than me. And I continue to learn from these consultants. Unfortunately, I sense in many of them a level of frustration and resignation that I've not seen previously. These consultants like the hospitalists often seem overwhelmed by patients dropped in the ER in the middle of the night. And sometimes families have unrealistic expectations that the doctor assigned to provide care cannot resolve. Defensive medicine is inevitable because the continuity of care of the trusted "family doctor" is not there.

There is an old saying that goes, "Doctor, lawyer, Indian chief; rich man, poor man, beggar man, thief." I feel blessed to be a doctor. I am convinced I'm doing the one thing I can do well in this life. Lots of people ask me how I'm doing these days and I reply that I'm sad about the passing of America and medical care. But, I then add, I'm coming to a sense of peace knowing that, as Paul once said, "I fought the good fight; I kept the faith and [will finish] the race."

October in Knoxville is wonderful – or as they say in Italian on my "bucket list" trip, bellissimo. About the time you get sick of one season, another comes along. I went out the other day and I felt it. The cooler, dryer weather made me think, "Fall is in the air." I've been on five continents and in more than forty countries, and though I like to travel, I'm always glad to come home to one of the most beautiful places in the world.

Recently, Becky and I spent several hours perimeter-spraying our mountain cabin. We do this to prevent infestation by lady bugs (whom I no longer consider "ladies"). I don't recall problems with these insects in the past. These bugs try to find a warm place for the winter and apparently my cabin is more desirable than the forest. I'm sympathetic, but swarms of invading lady bugs covering our walls are unacceptable. I step over creatures in the yard, but when they invade my space, it's war.

If you haven't seen them you must be blind. I'm referring to those ugly grey insects we call stink bugs. These Asian invaders began their infestation of America about fifteen years ago. They recently made it to Knoxville and seem to be everywhere. Bugs don't bother me, but hordes of them can be creepy. Recall, that even birds can be creepy if murderous like Alfred Hitchcock's, **The Birds**.

Most Sundays our family and friends often gather after church for Sunday lunch. The extent of the stink bug problem became real as a friend told us about her car wreck over Sunday lunch. She was backing out of her daughter's drive way, and the stink bug struck. The prehistoric looking pest dropped on her and she panicked, jumping out of the slowly rolling vehicle. She was knocked to the ground and the car actually ran over her foot! Amazingly, she wasn't seriously injured and as she rolled free she looked up to see her daughter flying to the rescue. Having just gotten out of the shower and clad only in a towel her daughter rushed to her Mom's aid. I listened in fascination as the daughter was described as diving toward the open car door, losing her cape in the process. "She's Batman!" I cried wiping back the tears of laughter.

I don't have any phobias, but several of my family members do. It's not uncommon for me to be pressed into service to remove a black snake from our yard or a praying mantis from around our barn. A phobia is an irrational fear of an object or a situation. Phobias include fear of animals, heights, insects or enclosed spaces (claustrophobia) such as MRI scanners or elevators. Sometimes severe anxiety can occur just by thinking about spiders, for instance, or hearing the word. Even injections or the anticipation of having blood drawn for laboratory testing can cause panic in some people. In the movie **Annie Hall**, Woody Allen had to save

Diane Keaton from a spider in her house. He ridiculed her until he confronted the "major" spider that was vanquished only with great drama and a broom.

The lifetime risk of developing a phobia is about twelve percent, though a bit higher in women than men. The condition tends to congregate in families, suggesting a genetic predilection influenced by an environmental stimulus or a traumatic event. In people with phobias, science has discovered over activation in certain areas of the brain known as the cingulate insula and the amygdala. With phobic stimuli these areas are activated and "negative emotional responses" result.

Some phobias are mild and just a nuisance, while others cause significant problems in daily life. Phobias often last a life time, but can be corrected by exposure-based treatment. Additionally, psychotherapy and medications like Prozac and Valium are helpful.

Most of us don't suffer from an irrational fear of things. I have a friend who totally freaks out if she sees a bug in her house. She wouldn't do well at our cabin where we sometimes find small scorpions or wasps. Logically, I ask, which is worse - an occasional insect or a house full of insecticides? But I don't suffer from phobias.

I feel sorry for folks with phobias who can't help their panic symptoms. The rest of us just want varmints to stay outside in nature where they belong. I've been known to carry granddaddy longlegs outside instead of swatting them. Even the occasional spider is tolerated because these arachnids prey upon and control insect populations. Go out early some morning this fall and notice the dew that reveals hundreds of spider webs. Without these eight-legged creatures we would be quickly over run by the six-legged ones (insects).

The threshold for me is infestation and safety. I step over bugs on the ground, but I'm currently battling fire ants that have sprung up all over Thistle Farm and recently stung my grandson, Oakley. I've declared war on these invaders from southern climes. And I've told the fruit flies that suddenly appear from nowhere or house flies that try and relocate from the horse manure strewn pastures that they will be swatted if they are found within the walls of our home.

Mostly I try and coexist with nature. However, I'm even less tolerant of the Big Stink that is emanating from Washington. Insects and other varmints like raccoons are just poor creatures trying to make it in the world. Obama and the Beltway Boys have chosen to stink up our country. Perhaps we need an industrial Orkin-ization of Washington, D.C.

The Gift of Touch - December 9, 2013

I've observed that as I get older I like change less. I'm not the first person to make this observation, but the pace of change is like no other in my lifetime. For the first twenty-five years of my life I didn't pay a lot of attention to politics or world events. I do remember the Cuban Missile Crisis because my parents took me out of school, and together we filled our bathtub with water in preparation for an imminent nuclear attack. And I remember the Vietnam Tet Offensive and Walter Cronkite reporting on the evening news that the Vietnam War was lost – and so it was.

During the last thirty-five years I've refocused my attention beyond my immediate horizon and conclude nothing is like it was when I came of age. In medical school I was taught the art of physical examination and diagnosis. Everyone studied the classic textbook, DeGowin's Diagnostic Examination, which I still own. I found my old friend as I was emptying my medical office book shelves. The notes in the margins were still there though faded by time.

In those days there were no CAT Scanners or panels of blood tests and you needed all your observational and clinical skills when you and your sick patient were alone in the middle of the night. There is a famous painting called **The Doctor** that hangs in the Tate Gallery in London. It depicts a house call, a sick child and things aren't going well. In the painting, the doctor sits like Rodin's sculpture, **The Thinker**, studying the child and hoping for inspiration. We now have wonderful diagnostic aids; I've been quick to correct young doctors too quick with the results of an echocardiogram (ultrasound of the heart) before describing their patient's heart sounds. My advice was to hone their clinical skills because sometimes that's all you've got in the middle of the night.

I have averaged 4000 patient visits a year for the last forty years. That's a lot of heart and belly examinations, and a huge comparative data base. Some years ago a patient presented to my office with what sounded like a viral syndrome and a secondary sinus infection. I did the necessary examination of her ears, nose and throat and listened to her heart and lungs. Because she was young she seldom saw me for care, choosing instead to see her OB-GYN. Perhaps it was a man's gut feeling (women have intuition) or maybe it was defensive medicine that made me examine her belly and discover the mass. Fortunately, her kidney cancer was discovered before it had spread and she was cured by surgery after her sinus infection was treated. The lesson – it takes so little to be thorough.

Over the years I have led numerous medical missions in Central America. In the mountains of Guatemala there are no CAT scanners or blood tests, and the only technology is your stethoscope. When I was in Medical School the TV program MASH was popular, especially with young medical students. When I went to medical school I thought I wanted to be a chest surgeon like Hawkeye Pierce who seemed to thrive in the crucible of trauma surgery. The Guatemalan bush is more primitive than Hawkeye's Korea of the 1950s, yet life and death is more real than that TV drama. My mantra and directive for my medical teams was that care is both a noun and a verb; however, the noun is only possible if the verb comes first. Every patient had the symbol of American technology (stethoscope) applied to their chest as a gift of touch and an instrument of care.

I sometimes feel that my stethoscope and my touch are no longer necessary in the New Order. These days, doctors complete patient records by checking electronic boxes on a computer screen. The record was perfect for the patient I saw last year. Her previous doctor's examination and Pap smear did not mention the mass in her belly now the size of a football. No one in the operating room believed the twenty-two pound tumor had materialized in the six months between "examinations." You be the judge of a system that focuses on record keeping rather than care.

I'll admit that I've quit looking at patient's retinas as part of my regular exam. Eye doctors do a much better job. However, I refuse to become so specialized that I pick an organ to treat rather than a patient. Does it matter that doctors these days don't routinely check their patients for hernias? I guess we should wait till a patient reports a bulge in the groin, complains of pain or presents with an obstructed bowel. Perhaps the thorough exam I've done on patients all my life is not necessary or "cost effective" in the New Order. But how can you measure care or the value of touch? Some say care is best measured by a well-documented medical record with all the appropriate screening tests ordered by surrogates. I say it is a verb that comes from the heart, and is measured by a hand that is held and a pulse that is felt. Emily Dickinson once wrote, "Hope is the thing with feathers – that perches in the soul…" I might substitute the word care for hope.

Two thousand years ago The Master said, "It is not the healthy who need a doctor, but the sick" (Matthew 9:12). The New Order has turned the wisdom of the ages upside down and has institutionalized testing in the hopes of eventually reducing costs. What happens when all the money goes for expensive and mandated screening tests, and there's nothing left over for the care of the old or sick? Perhaps someone in the media should ask Obama and the Beltway Boys.

Each week I sit down to write because it gives me joy, and as I do so I thank Mr. Steve Hunley, my publisher, for giving me my voice. That's writer's lingo for an outlet for my creative muse. Ten years ago he decided that Knoxville needed an alternative to our daily newspaper and the Knoxville Focus was born.

Humans are time oriented creatures. We exist in this moment, but consider the past and the future. We celebrate birthdays, anniversaries and look forward to special events that shake us out of the doldrums and our routines. I have a friend who is a Jehovah Witness. He tells me that his denomination doesn't acknowledge special days, even Christmas. This devout Christian maintains that every day is a special day. I understand what he's saying because I wake up each morning thanking the Master that I'm able to re-boot my brain-computer and enjoy another day of life. The psalmist once said, "This is the day the Lord hath made. Let us rejoice and be glad in it."

Not to criticize my friend, but I love "special" days and moments. I think humans occasionally need a break and to occasionally "kick it up a notch," as Emeril would say. So, as Bill and Ted said in their **Excellent Adventure** "Party on, Dudes" of the Focus, and Happy Tenth Anniversary!

I've thought about starting a blog as friends have urged me to do. However, I'm fiercely loyal to the Focus and writing is my avocation not my vocation. I wonder if writing to make a living would commercialize my message. I never wrote anything beyond college assignments until 2001, when a friend challenged me to begin spiritual journaling. Perhaps Mr. Hunley noticed in me something I hadn't been aware of, because I'm a teacher at heart. Now, my teaching is extended beyond my patients because I'm told the Focus is read in all fifty states and in seventy countries.

Do humans have an essence beyond our flesh and blood or the obvious? I happen to believe that we are more than the sum of our parts. I read an article some years ago that purported to have calculated the value of chemicals in a human body. It was chump change. Man is obviously more than his renderings. In fact, all life is wondrous even if we occasionally take it for granted. A man named Protagoras once said, "Man is the measure of all things." I believe that is hubris (arrogant pride)! Even with all our knowledge and science we can't create a single microbe. "We are fearfully and wonderfully made," said the Psalmist. And we were gifted reason which we believe makes us special as the highest life form on this Earth and perhaps anywhere in the Cosmos. I personally doubt that we are alone in the universe. I explored that perspective in my novel, **Epiphany.** In his book "**The Victory of Reason**" professor Rodney Stark makes the point that God is rational and can be known by his rational creation, man. Read Isaiah 1:17-18, if you need another reference point for this assertion.

The educator David McCullough, Jr. (son of the author and historian David McCullough) recently said at a commencement address that none of us is special – everyone is. This assertion seems to go against the grain in our politically correct world of 2012, where children are often coddled. I often wonder what my life would have been like if I had never been challenged or failed. I didn't always win a trophy growing up. With hard work and opportunity I was accepted into medical school and I began a blessed life. Now, I wonder what the next phase of my life will be as a writer and educator and a celebrant of the way, the truth and the life.

Take my word for it, writing honestly is risky. When I first penned my thoughts for public consumption it felt like being naked in a crowd. And yet there was a blessing awaiting me I had never imagined. At my first book signing I thought a few friends and fellow parishioners might attend, but I was overwhelmed when crowds of friends and patients came to support me. As I signed books I had the image of attending my own funeral and seeing how many lives I had touched.

I've come to realize that we are all God's touch in a needy world. We are in fact special.

I am constantly amazed by what women carry in their pocketbooks. In fact, I think the descriptive phrase "pocketbook" for this accessory is a misnomer because there is no way you could get all that junk in a pocket. Perhaps we should always use the term handbags, even though they sometimes are so large and heavy that they remind me more of backpacks or saddlebags.

Some of my frailest patients carry the largest bags, containing enough gear for a camping trip. It's surprising that the geriatric literature has not described an increased risk of falls occasioned by tripping over handbags left beside chairs or by hoisting these satchels to the shoulder. Obviously, a twenty-pound bag hung over the shoulder with a strap will shift one's center of gravity and might further stress an already precarious balance problem.

Men don't understand things that a woman might need at a moment's notice – like the sunglasses my wife suddenly needed as we drove west one afternoon. As I rustled through her "pocketbook" looking and feeling around for her elusive sunglasses, I came upon a hammer. Becky is the "Handy Mam" in our household, enabling me to practice medicine and be contemplative; but a hammer in a handbag is ridiculous. And so was the twenty-foot metal tape measure I also found at the bottom of her bag, which I observed sarcastically that no girl should leave home without.

However, the prize goes to my ninety-five year old mother-in-law. About six months ago we were riding in the car and the topic of Obama's missing birth certificate came up. Joanna was puzzled by the president's difficulty finding his birth certificate because she had hers right there in her pocketbook! You can't make this kind of stuff up, folks.

After handing Becky her sunglasses with a chuckle, I thought about how I had used sight, touch, and hearing to penetrate the deep and cluttered environs of her clutch, aka purse. I was even treated to the familiar smell of her perfume as I prowled among her effects. Fortunately, all my senses remain intact though my sense of smell pales in comparison to Becky's. In general, a man's sense of smell is less than a woman's, and everyone's sense of smell declines as we age. Taste is another of our senses and is highly dependent upon smell; and both suffer with aging or a cold.

Hearing also declines as we age and can make older persons seem less sharp than they actually are. The ear also is a sensory organ for balance, and dysfunction of the inner ear causes vertigo, a spinning sensation. Most people have experienced the unsteadiness of vertigo that some describe as a sense of movement. While it may occur from excessive celebration on New Year's Eve or brain diseases, vertigo usually occurs from stones in the middle ear (you read this correctly) or irritation of the sensory cells within the inner ear. Vertigo is treatable and often resolves, hopefully before it throws you to the floor and breaks your hip.

Another sensory problem of aging is neuropathy – nerve damage – associated with a loss of sensation in the toes and feet. As I sit here, I can feel my toes and sense where and how they touch the ground. Specialized sensory organelles in the skin send signals to the brain through the spinal cord which we take for granted until they are damaged. Then we try to compensate by watching our feet as we walk. You may have noticed your grandfather with diabetes shorten his step, lift his feet higher and gaze downward at his feet to make sure of his step.

Unfortunately, compensation can only go so far, especially because our vision changes as we age. One eye is often stronger than the other, and older eyes are often corrected with bifocals and trifocals. Together these can alter depth perception especially with downward gazing. I'll never forget the first time I descended the hospital stairway with my first set of bifocals and almost traded my stethoscope for a cast on my leg.

They say that the eye is the window of the soul and I imagine that the loss of sight would be most devastating. Scientists can elegantly describe how light stimulates the photoreceptors of the retina and then explain how electro-chemical signals are sent to the brain for interpretation. Picture a tennis ball with a hole cut out of the front. If you were to look through the hole you'd see the back of the tennis ball just as you would the back of the eye and the retina if you looked through the pupil – so much for anatomy and physiology.

The Romantic era of the 1800s replaced the Classical era with a new perspective. Observational facts were trumped by a sense of the sublime. The Classical Enlightenment age thinkers emphasized the science of light and observational truth. The Romantics said they preferred to marvel at the beauty of a sunset.

As a post-modern 21st century philosopher, I ask, why must I choose between the beauty of scientific understanding and the wonder that it produces in my soul?

I admire the prose of Rick Bragg, the southern writer and author of several books as well as a monthly column in Southern Living magazine. Perhaps if I had followed a different time line I might have had a writing vocation rather than a mid-life avocation. But who knows. I feel blessed to have a career in medicine that continues to fascinate me.

I managed to make it to the Knoxville Pops concert last week despite my recent *GIs*. Our entire family has been beset with this affliction, also known as gastrointestinal upset, which has recently been terrorizing the Knoxville community. Our version encompassed diarrhea with abdominal cramps, as well as the ever-popular nausea with occasional vomiting. I told our symphony group not to shake my hand or stand too close to me as I had just been released from *quarantine*. I garnered considerable empathy from my friends because most had experienced the "bug-prep," which I told them had sufficiently prepped me for a colonoscopy, though my doctor had not scheduled one.

I think it's good to occasionally move outside your comfort zone and expand your horizons. Last year I attended a Knoxville Pops Concert featuring the group ABBA, whose music I do not care for. Nonetheless, I went and received more than I bargained for as I learned about music and speech patterns that translated into a story for the Focus. Similarly, you should never miss an issue of the Focus because you never know what I'll say or you what you might.

Last week's concert featuring the Cirque de la Symphonie again challenged me because I don't particularly like circus acts or clowns. Seinfeld's TV character, Kramer, is afraid of clowns, and my grandson, Oakley, views the "tickle monster" with a similar mixture of delight and dread. The Cirque de la Symphonie is unusual in that it is the only Cirque du Soleil company that performs with symphony orchestras. There is a certain shtick associated with the Cirque du Soleil brand that I best describe as edgy artistic athleticism.

Europeans, and especially the French, view the world differently than most Americans – except perhaps John Kerry. I was <u>beguiled</u> by the Cirque's unique interpretation of movement and dance, counterpoised with strength and balance, set to magnificent classical music selections played by our outstanding Knoxville Symphony. Over the years I've been challenged by readers who tell me I don't have credentials to comment outside the field of medicine. I've respectfully responded with, "Hogwash." This column is after all an opinion column.

Generally I prefer opera to the symphony because there is just more eye-candy with opera. In opera there are costumes, dance and of course operatic drama accompanied by beautiful music with sublime vocalization. The classical era composer, Mozart, felt that the human voice was the acme of music. He said nowhere else can multiple different melodies be sung and yet work together. An example is the quartet in act 2 of Verdi's Rigoletto. Mozart never experienced Cirque du Soleil, but if the movie **Amadeus** provides any insight into the prodigy's temperament, he would have loved it.

No, this column doesn't have a medical focus unless you recall your last bout of Montezuma's revenge or the pleasure of a colonoscopy prep. I've considered abandoning medical themes all together, but there's still too much doctor in me to do an about face at sixty-three. I've already been through several course corrections in my journey. I began my writing career at fifty with daily spiritual *journaling*. How interesting that Mr. Webster doesn't recognize this word. English is a living language that changes over time. Who would have imagined a mouse as something other than a pest scurrying across your counter twenty years ago? Apparently, Mr. Webster also isn't aware of the nonce word "sniglets," words that are not in the dictionary, but should be.

Not infrequently patients ask me if I do surgery. Often my reply is to point to the replica of Rodin's *The Thinker* on my desk and quip, "No, I'm a *thinker*, not a cutter." This is meant to be tongue-in-cheek humor, not a slam of my surgical colleagues. Modern internists and surgeons are trained in the scientific method and gravitate to either a contemplative or a more hands-on therapeutic mode. Historically, doctors were university men, but after the Council of Tours in 1163, they were banned from doing surgery.

The surgical discipline extends back to Galen, physician of the Roman emperors and gladiators. In the Middle Ages surgery was associated with barbers who were capable of doing simple operations like bloodletting, dental extractions and lancing boils. I have no illusion that an internist would be as valuable today as a surgeon if our civilization suffered a meltdown. After all, an internist would not be as valuable without a CT scanner or a diagnostic lab.

I first heard the term sawbones in TV westerns. Doctors were so named because they could saw off a limb rapidly enough to save their patients. When I went to medical school I thought I wanted to be a chest surgeon like Hawkeye Pierce on *MASH*. During medical school I gained extra experience working as a "suture student" sewing up members of the local "Knife and Bottle" club who met regularly on Friday and Saturday nights in Memphis. This vision of the underbelly of life cured me of the perceived glory amidst the gore.

The John Gaston Hospital of Memphis where I trained no longer exists, but it was a big inner city hospital like Charity hospital in New Orleans and Bellevue in New York. I was subjected to a *sink or swim* training style that taught me how to maintain my head in a crisis. I've delivered three dozen babies, resuscitated patients when an EKG machine shorted out and caught on fire, and spent long nights adjusting ventilator settings of comatose patients. I tell patients I could take out their appendix in an emergency, but they might not be quite the same afterwards.

Recently, I sat by the Atlantic Ocean and reflected on my life and career. Contemplative moments come to lots of people at the beach. As I sat there I watched the relentless pounding of the surf as it broke down shells to ever smaller bits producing the beaches of the world. I'm told that there are more stars in the universe than grains of sand on all the beaches of the world, but that's another story line.

I had a similar vision of recycled life as I helped my family operate a portable sawmill to cut our pine trees and cedars into planks for the barn raising. I had never experienced a sawmill at work. As the logs were cut by the band saw, the sawdust piled up. It was golden white from the pines and purple from the cedars. However, the vivid colors faded as they mixed just as the multicolored shells when pulverized become white sand.

"No man is an island," said John Donne. We are all "a part of the main." Those sea creatures lived and died and then gave their shells back as sand. Our pines and cedars are being recycled too. We will waste nothing. The boards will be siding for the barn. The shavings will be processed with a chipper and used on the floors of the horse stalls. And everything will return to the earth from which it came and be used again.

I lost another friend this week. He was a stalwart in our church, and he was full of life and vigor at eighty-four. He dropped dead getting his paper the other morning, but I believe only the atoms of his body will be recycled. His essence has moved on, and his *color* has only intensified.

You realize that humans see only a limited part of the electromagnetic spectrum. Now we see "dimly as in a mirror," Paul said. My friend now sees fully, and resides as part of the entire spectrum of Light.

I've yet to experience *writer's block* – the condition where writers run out of things to say. Every week a story seems to present itself, but I wondered if this week would be an exception. I was concerned because my anxious mood was affecting my creative muse. For the non-literary folks, a muse is akin to the tiny beings that stood on the shoulders of Looney Tune cartoon characters and whispered into their ears. A more Olympian vision was that of the ancient Greeks who imagined nine goddesses that motivated poets and artists.

Wisdom writings observe that we'll always have something to worry about, and the worry doesn't do us a lot of good. It's much better to focus on the Transcendent than to be consumed with worry about the present. It's easy for me to get torqued when I focus on my immediate struggles, past mistakes or when I worry about tomorrow. Last Saturday I remember awakening and being at peace for about two hours. What a blessing.

The dead of winter is a troublesome time for a lot of people. I think the only thing good about February is that it's short. There's even a medical/psychiatric condition called SAD, or seasonal affective disorder, which is associated with a deficiency of sunlight during the winter months. The physiology of this problem is thought to occur because the paucity of sunlight causes less stimulation of the pineal gland and a disruption of melatonin production. You can picture the location of this tiny hormone-producing organ in the center of your head by placing your finger on the bridge of your nose and pointing toward the back of your skull. The pituitary gland regulates our body rhythms and sleep. In some persons the lack of sunlight and melatonin production is associated with clinical depression. Jet lag is a condition which occurs with travel across multiple time zones. It is associated with melatonin fluctuations and alteration in bodily rhythms.

Some years ago a friend told me a proverb attributed to a man named Jos Mart who said you should, "Plant a tree, write a book and have a son." Well, I've written a book – I'm working on a second – I've raised two daughters with my wife and one daughter is pregnant with a son. And today I planted an orchard.

The *Bucket List* is a wonderful movie where Jack Nicholson and Morgan Freeman try to experience all their dreams before they die. Well, I'm not dying and I'm still planning for the future. I hope my fruit trees will survive our pitiful south Knoxville soil and eventually produce fruit. Someone once said that we should plant a tree that we'll never expect to see mature. What a noble and selfless attitude. This seems lost in our often solipsistic (word for the week) modern world.

187

I wrote an essay some weeks ago entitled *Entropy*. You should go to the knoxfocus. com website and read this story which generated more responses than any I've written in the last four years. This principle of the universe (entropy) is the reason time processes forward rather than in reverse. This may sound like a ridiculous statement because everyone experiences linear time with a past, present and a future. Actually, this notion of a timeline is a western concept. People in other cultures envision time as circular and call it the *wheel of life*. The writer's of the *Lion King* redacted (second word of the week) this concept as the *circle of life* and made a fortune.

What if time is an infinity of present moments? I love the movie *Ground Hog Day* with Bill Murray. In this campy movie, the protagonist is caught in a recurring segment of time until he learns humility and empathy. The great 20th century apologist (third word of the week) for Christianity, C. S. Lewis, posited that God exists out of space and time which governs us mortals.

In his book **The Gift of the Jews**, Thomas Cahill posits that our western sense of time began when God interacted with humans and established our time line. However, if Lewis is right then God perceives us outside our sense of time. Past and future may actually merge with an infinity of present moments in the presence of God.

Well, that's certainly abstruse (fourth word of the week). I just love finding the right word for a thought! I find that I'm most alive when I write or journal. When writing I sense inspiration and direction from the greatest Muse, the Architect of all that is. He is the Maker of trees and Fergusons and all space and time.

So what is required of me as I traverse this wondrous reality called life? The prophet Micah said it best, "Do justice, love mercy and walk humbly with your God"; and plant trees along the way.

My patient was deathly sick when I saw him in the intensive care unit (ICU). He was on a ventilator and thankfully still unconscious after emergency surgery to remove his gangrenous appendix that had ruptured. It's amazing how someone can get so sick so quickly; I had seen Mr. W the week before for his annual physical and now his "clean bill of health" was a moot point.

Actually, Mr. W has medical problems commensurate with his 75 years, but these didn't slow him down as he sailed through hip surgery earlier in the year. Now, he'd need all his reserves and a lot of luck to survive. A ruptured bowel that empties the equivalent of sewage into the abdominal cavity is a mortal wound without modern medical care.

Families are often shocked when they see their loved ones in the ICU. This most often happens after coronary bypass surgery (CABG). In order to graft a vascular bypass around blockages in diseased heart arteries, the surgeons and anesthesiologists divert the circulation and stop the heart. Your brain and body can't be deprived of oxygen and nutrients so doctors rely on an artificial pump to sustain life during the operation.

It's a complicated procedure to put someone to sleep and connect them to the heart-lung machine. Once connected, the heart is cooled and stopped with an electrical shock which immobilizes the heart so the surgeon can do his delicate repair work. After completing the vascular bypass (detour) around the blocked arteries, the heart is then re-warmed and shocked back into pumping. The patient is disconnected from the bypass machine, the chest is wired back together and anesthesia is discontinued. It's brutal work and amazing that patients do so well. I suspect they improve because critical deficiencies are corrected and patients literally "pink up" with improved heart function. By the next morning they're often up in a chair.

Mr. W's situation was more tenuous. The crusty ICU nurses had seen it all before – emergency surgery and kidney failure in an older body with limited reserves. Their raised eyebrows told me what everyone knew: Mr. W wasn't going to make it even though we would exert heroic efforts to save him. I discussed the situation with his wife and left the details of his ventilator management to the critical care physician and fluid therapy to his kidney specialist. In years past I would have been the doctor in charge of his frightful condition, but how often does an internist/ geriatrician have such a sick patient? Perhaps twice a year, and those who do this kind of specialized work on a daily basis are now more capable than me.

I've read about doctors in past eras and their almost prescient abilities of prognostication. Perhaps *mortal wounds* were so named because so little could be done without operating rooms, antibiotics and therapies to correct shock. And I suspect a hundred years from now someone will read in a book and marvel at how anyone could survive the *barbaric* treatments we call modern medicine today.

And yet in spite of the naysayers, Mr. W improved. He made a liar out of the statistics that said he was doomed and that we should not be wasting valuable societal resources in such a futile effort. You've heard those statistics, where a lot of money is spent in the last year of someone's life. I believe these are skewed statistics because expense is calculated from the person's time of death. If the person survives, the bean counter's expense curve is skewed.

Mr. W's care would not be counted with the expenses of dying because he was weaned from the ventilator, his kidneys recovered and he woke up to see me leaning over him listening to his heart and lungs. He even shocked the nurses when he asked them to help him take a little walk. Imagine an ICU nurse's reaction when a patient asks them to *take a hike*!

We don't know why some people do well and others don't. Undoubtedly, good doctors and excellent nursing care help, but there are other intangibles like the life force that beats hard in some and less so in others. I'll admit, sometimes it's luck. Sometimes we classify it as a mystery.

"I'm glad you're feeling better, Mr. W," as I listened to his lungs the next day. I told him we'd all been worried about him. Then I quipped to lighten the situation, "I've heard that if the Lord gets you right He'll take you home." With a wink I added, "Apparently, He's decided to send you back for some *remedial work*." Mr. W just smiled.

Is there such a thing as right or wrong? Do people know what's right or have a standard? Perhaps they've just forgotten and need reassurance and encouragement to "speak the truth in love."

Sometimes in my medical practice I feel like a cheerleader at a pep rally. I try not to lecture, but it's hard because I grew up with the "encouraging words" of my ex-military father. I suspect people know what they should do to maximize their health; it's just tough to diet and avoid tobacco and drugs. Perhaps my patients just want me to pull a rabbit out of the hat. Modern medicine does seem to border on magic sometimes, but most of the time it's just common sense and applied science.

Lately, I've been thinking about ontological questions. Say what? **Ontology** is the study of being. In other words, the reason we are the way we are. The 18th century French philosopher Henri Rousseau said that we are born with a blank slate called the *tabula rasa*. And he said that society corrupts the otherwise *noble savage*. Rousseau believed that if people were educated and provided sufficient food a utopian society would occur. It hasn't worked in America or anywhere else. Americans have plenty of educational opportunities and enough food to make two thirds of us overweight or obese – so much for Rousseau's philosophy.

Luminaries such as Socrates, Sophocles, Cicero, St. Paul, Thomas Aquinas, John Locke and Thomas Jefferson all had a different take on the question of being and the human condition. Jefferson's synthesis of Natural Law theory says it best; "We hold these Truths to be self-evident, that all Men are created equal, that they are endowed by their Creator with certain unalienable Rights, that among these are Life, Liberty, and the pursuit of Happiness – That to secure these Rights, Governments are instituted among Men, deriving their just Powers from the Consent of the Governed..." I've always been intrigued by Jefferson's use of capitals. Was this for emphasis or was he acknowledging the Divine source of "rights" that makes us what we are?

In America we are now engaged in a great debate asking whether the State or the Spirit is the prime motivator of humanity and *right*. John Adams once asked if we were a country of laws or men. That question is again relevant these days. Two thousand years ago the nascent Christian church practiced **koinonia**, incompletely translated as fellowship because this was more than Wednesday night fellowship and potluck supper. The folks in Acts truly shared all they had.

Controversy arose about a hundred years ago with the reinterpretation of the koinonia philosophy in America. Two perspectives emerged among Christian groups. One group held that koinonia was a *social gospel* where the Church was called to aid the least fortunate and change the world. The other group's interpretation emphasized the transformation of the individual through the gospel's message. It was the new man who then went forward to change the world. I personally identify with both perspectives, but the sectarian debate continues and even extends to the philosophies of our two dominant political parties.

The ancient Greeks ascribed to what we now call the cardinal virtues or right behavior. They said that a society could be built on courage, common sense, moderation and justice. Unfortunately, this only works in a society with the same backgrounds and standards. And even then, situational ethics can take over as in Victor Hugo's story *Les Miserables*.

Humans need a standard by which to measure themselves. If I tell someone to measure a door frame and they report to me that it's thirty-six inches, I trust they've used a yardstick and not a meter stick. Otherwise, we're in real trouble. NASA made this error some years ago. St. Paul articulated a higher level of standards or morality with what we now call the theological virtues of faith, hope and love.

I was getting a cup of coffee last Saturday in the Doctor's lounge when I heard several *older* colleagues grumbling about being on-call and how things have changed. It's natural to feel that your cohort has it tougher than the rising generation. However, I was struck by their observation that the new generation of doctors is more focused on lifestyle issues rather than the "calling" of medicine. It made me reconsider the notion of *right* and who I would want to be in charge of my care. I read once that the definition of a professional is a person whose work and life are inseparable. I may be at the beach, but I'm still a doctor to my core.

Hippocrates was a physician most known to us for his Hippocratic Oath. There's a lot in his now famous oath that isn't germane for modern times, but his perspective that a doctor is *called* to do his best for the patient he serves has been the mantra of medicine for thousands of years. The world is changing and the emphasis of the new order is for doctors to refocus on cost-effective *herd* management rather than on the one lost sheep that wanders off from the ninety-nine and shows up in the ER.

I'm not sure what's going to happen, and this seems to be a common concern these days among doctors and citizens. What I do know is that I side with the philosophy of the Master, and do my best and my duty to help one sheep at a time.

A woman recently wrote me to say that I should confine my writings to medical issues and not speak of history, philosophy or politics. Apparently, she didn't have any problems with my frequent mention of religion, the Spirit, the Master or God. I told her I write about what's on my mind and heart at the moment, and I can't write or speak disingenuously. I'd probably be a lousy politician. I told her she is free to read my column or not, but I rejected her assertion that my words were "divisive" for the country. And though the Knoxville Focus has a substantial circulation, I doubt my words have national significance.

These days we often hear descriptive adjectives such as **divisive** or **hateful** in the description of someone's position. You need to understand that these terms are used to dismiss or diminish another's opinion. In other words, the rhetorical use of certain words undercuts any substance of the opposing argument. This rhetorical technique is called an **ad hominem** attack on the person rather than his argument. By denigrating the person, his words are made irrelevant. Another way to misrepresent someone's opinion is the **straw man** fallacy. An example of this rhetorical trick is to say that Mitt Romney hates women because he does not support taxpayer funded condoms.

I write a lot these days about democracy and the direction of our country. The ancient Greek statesman Pericles once opined that citizens who say they're minding their own business rather than participating in the affairs of the polis (the state), actually have no business there at all. So you see **all** engaged citizens are important and necessary in a democracy. I challenged my reader, a liberal philosoph, to welcome diverse opinions. Unfortunately, she seems to be illiberal as she attempts to silence me. And I write about history to remind people that "Those who cannot remember the past are condemned to repeat it" (George Santayana).

As a trained observer of human behavior I frequently ask myself why people behave as they do. I'm a fan of the **Seinfeld** sitcom, and the quote by George Costanza seems relevant today. He said, "It's not a lie if you believe it." Could this be why our politicians lie to us? Have they convinced themselves of the events in Benghazi, Libya? Or is this tragedy just incompetence and an ill-conceived foreign policy? Perhaps it is politically mediated deception of the American people to cover up for past political rhetoric.

"These are the times that try men's souls," said Thomas Paine in December 1776 when things seemed really bad for our nascent country. Our lot is much better than those Continental soldiers who shivered in the forest avoiding the more powerful and better equipped British Redcoats pursuing them. And radical Islamists aren't shooting at me or trying to blow up my friends in the adjacent Humvee. Yet, our nation and the free world are in real trouble, so as a citizen I must speak out. Smiley faces and Kumbaya diplomacy only puts us in greater jeopardy.

The 20th century Christian apologist C. S. Lewis said, "We live in enemy territory." He was speaking of our "fallen world" that is subject to the malevolent forces of darkness. However, I believe there may be non-spiritual tyrannies currently operative that strive to enslave free men and make them subservient to an all-powerful state run by the elite few. Some would say I am foolish and that our huge Federal Government is our friend and will take care of us. I admit that I trust in Providence, my family and friends and my neighbors more than the State.

These days I revel in caring for my grandson and watching him grow and discover the world around him. I watch his eyes as he takes in his surroundings. Everything is new to him; not like adults who've seen it all before and have become jaded. We remember little of our first years, but the foundations of our minds and spirit are laid like footers for a building. Once the building goes up we no longer see the foundation, but it's there.

My job is to make sure Oakley has a firm foundation and is nurtured and protected. My job is to make sure he has the opportunity for "life, liberty and the pursuit of happiness." That's what this election is all about. And when it's over and the country is saved, I'll go back to the peaceful pursuit of medicine. We all need a rest!

A Natal Star - March 9, 2015

A new star has appeared in the heavens, and nothing will be the same for us again.

Astrology is a pseudoscience which believes the orientation of heavenly bodies when we're born determines our character and personality. I'm a scientist and I don't believe in astrology. However, seeing Josie, my newborn granddaughter, causes me to question empirical science. This tiny "earthly star" melts my heart and drives me to my proverbial knees. The Wise Men were astrologers and followed the natal star of the Christ child to Bethlehem. They traveled more than a thousand miles to kneel before a baby who would change the world. My daughter's hospital room was just across town and far grander than a manger. None the less, I imagined the manger scene as family and friends (shepherds of children), and sometimes wise men, all paid homage to this new beacon of hope.

Josie took her own sweet time, arriving almost a week "late" by the doctor's calculations. Modern medicine does a much better job predicting due-dates than in times past. Formerly, our calculations were extrapolated from the mother's last menstrual period. Now, the baby's intrauterine development and milestones can be accurately observed with sophisticated ultrasound technology. Obstetricians can even measure declining amniotic fluid levels which can signify an "overdue" baby, raising the risk of fetal distress.

I must confess, the spiritual side of me now chafes at the term fetus. I rarely look up medical definitions these days, but I recently did so. Science defines a human embryo as gestational life during the first two months after conception. Then the medical term fetus is used to define a human organism from three months till birth. Folks, Josie was a baby the day before she was born, and the weeks and even months before she was delivered.

I understand that in the past an unborn was considered not human. And the ancient Greeks held that male children before manhood (and all women) were sub-human. Even Ezekiel Emanuel (Rom's brother) doesn't make this claim, though some today feel more comfortable aborting a fetus instead of an intrauterine baby.

When does human life begin? Is it at the moment of conception when there is a full complement of human DNA? Or is the "embryo" only proto-life, destined to become fully human sometime later – perhaps after the teenage years? Until such time as scientists, philosophers, theologians and ethicists can define the point of transition when proto-life becomes a sentient human being with God given rights, I must side with the sacredness of life.

We come from water. Science holds that life on earth began in the sea or its tide pools. I thought about Josie, recently afloat in a salty sea just like my ancient ancestors – and me sixty-four years ago. In the first trimester of life (first three months) organs like the brain are formed and the heart begins to beat and pump blood. The organs and systems undergo further development in the second three months of intrauterine life. The last trimester is largely a time of growing strong enough to survive outside the womb's warm and nurturing salt sea. I wondered what Josie was thinking when her mother's water broke and labor contractions forced her ashore into a "brave new world." From the delivery-room picture of her furrowed brow, she might say that "it's been a rough day."

Since we come from water, it has acquired much symbolism. An obvious example is Christian baptism. Interestingly, baptism predates Christianity. In Judaism, mikvah denotes the practice of ritual immersion which was integral to prayer and study. I find it noteworthy that Jesus began his ministry with baptism in the Jordan River by John the Baptizer.

Water covers 71% of the earth's surface and is necessary for life, at least as we know it. Scientists continue to look for signs of water on Mars as they search for life beyond the earth. We wonder if we're alone in the universe, comprised of more than 10^{18} suns/stars besides our own. This represents a vast sea of possibilities, where planets with water and life might exist. We've found more than 700 exoplanets circling distant suns, but none of these are like our earth as famously photographed by Apollo 8 in 1968 (Google Earthrise). Science fiction has speculated that life might be constructed on a silicon base rather than carbon, or float like gas bags in a hydrogen/helium atmosphere like Jupiter's. The SETI project, described in the movie **Contact**, searched for radio signals of life elsewhere in the cosmos, but to date we remain alone. (Most of us reject notions of aliens at Roswell, New Mexico.)

Our Josie-girl literally glows like a star in the heavens. John Boehner might be proud of Josie's "tan," but he'd be misguided. Josie has the soft glow of neonatal jaundice. The liver of newborns is still immature and often has difficulty clearing the metabolites of red blood cells (heme). Furthermore, neonates have more red cells than adults, and their fetal hemoglobin doesn't last as long as the mature oxygen-carrying hemoglobin infants soon acquire. Together these cause a greater load on the newborn liver. And surprisingly, breast feeding can contribute to elevated bilirubin levels and neonatal jaundice because an unknown factor in breast milk causes increased intestinal absorption of bile pigments derived from heme breakdown.

We tend to take pregnancy with labor and delivery for granted, and usually things go well. However, we shouldn't ignore the potential for complications which can be sudden and dramatic. I've observed that labor and delivery can transform a healthy young person into a life threatening condition – in the blink of an eye. I may be offending some, but I believe an experienced obstetrician and modern care are important for a safe delivery and monitoring fragile newborns afterwards.

I think pictures are sometimes worth more than words, especially when those words come from a "sometimes wise" man. So I will step back and introduce you to the "Star." World, this is Ms. Josie Johnson. Protect her with your prayers that she may grow up to be a seeker of wisdom and the stars.

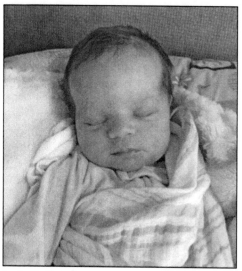

Josie Emily Johnson
(born 03.03.2015)

It seems only fitting that the last essay in this collection should be the first of a new year and a new direction.

The New Look - January 10, 2015

Winter's cold had finally come and I needed my heavy coat. I expected to find it pushed to the back of our closet by other season's garb. I never expected to find, instead, the coat of a bygone era. My white hospital lab coat, now relegated to the back of the closet, was where I left it, along with my traditional medical practice, December 31, 2013. That date marked, for me, a changing of the guard and a change of the garb.

There is a time honored tradition in medical school called the White Coat Ceremony. When students become juniors, having passed all their basic science courses they are awarded their first white coat. And even though it is a short version of a real doctor's (RD) coat, it is nonetheless a coveted rite of passage and the gateway to membership in an elite group.

Seeing my old hospital coat, with one of my stethoscopes still in the pocket, brought back memories of a career spanning four decades. I now tell people, "I'm not retired," when they ask me if I'm enjoying retirement. I love Mark Twain's often dry humor. He once quipped that "The news of my death has been greatly exaggerated." The same can be said of this doctor who has rediscovered the joy of practicing medicine again, outside the disintegrating modern "industrial-medical complex." I now tell people I'm semi-retired and I practice concierge medicine. I no longer work for anyone other than my patients. Now, I've traded the longer version of a M.D.'s white hospital coat for the doctor's bag given to me at my graduation from medical school in 1975.

For me life is certainly different as this New Year dawns. Looking back, I can honestly say that leaving the "system" was my destiny. It took two years of soul searching and a leap of faith – born of desperation – to walk away from all I had worked for since I was eighteen years old. Only later did I discover that concierge medicine as a new business venture would be a godsend. I especially identify with this word, because I believe in a deterministic universe with a purpose and plan and an Intelligent Designer. His plan is often mysterious, perhaps because His ways are not our ways (Isaiah 55:8). Yet life and Creation are majestic.

Making house calls in my truck is certainly different than seeing patients in a medical office or in a hospital surrounded by technology, support staff and readily available colleagues when consultation is necessary. Perhaps medical missionary work in Central America, far from technology, honed my diagnostic skills and now allows me to listen, observe and make decisions without a CAT scan. Don't get the wrong impression; I'm not a medical troglodyte. I still order simple and complex tests on my patients. However, we should all question whether we do too much testing, take too many pills, and apply too little common sense these days. At this point in my life, I've come to understand what is right, and what is not.

Forgive me for getting a bit preachy and philosophical. You can take the boy out of the white coat, but not the white coat out of the boy. A few light hearted observations of concierge medicine might afford a smile. Ladies especially may empathize with a professional patient of mine who chose to come to my home for her annual exam because she didn't "want to clean her house for my visit!" When my medical group broke up, we divided the medical equipment and found there was an extra exam table which I took home and put in my library. My resourceful wife was able to balance "form and function" by placing an attractive screen in front of the otherwise out of place sterile table. Now, my grandson hardly notices the table when he naps in his bed on the other side of the screen.

Few would argue that, in general, men are less modest than women. I once did a *delicate* examination on a patient in his living room. Experience is a great teacher and while I was *probing* I noticed that the drapes were open. I hoped that the neighbors weren't curious about the red truck in the driveway, and weren't scanning the windows. I won't make that mistake again. Similarly, another patient was very concerned about a new lump she had discovered in her breast. As I was examining her, it suddenly occurred to me how awkward it might appear if her husband were to chance upon his wife and me. Ordinarily, in my concierge medical practice, women maintain their relationship with their OB-Gyn, and in my former office practice I always had a female attendant during "sensitive" female examinations. Perhaps someone might explain to me why women physicians are not similarly required to have an attendant when examining their male patients.

Another milestone passed with the exit of 2014. On average I saw four thousand patients a year for almost forty years, and was never sued for malpractice. This is very unusual. Perhaps I was lucky; perhaps I was competent. I suspect it was more because my patients knew that I cared for them. We spent quality time with each other and our relationships transcended standard medical care. Many of my former patients remain my friends. I've made medical mistakes, but not because of a detached or reckless attitude. And friends, more often than not, forgive each other.

We hear much these days about "best" medical practices judged by arbitrary surrogates like blood pressure readings, Hemoglobin A1c levels (diabetic control) or what percentage of a doctor's patients went for mammograms. Perhaps these indirect markers are easier for bean counters to assess than quality time spent with a patient.

A recent essay in JAMA (Journal of the American Medical Association) asked the question, "Who determines physician effectiveness?" My *a priori* bias was challenged when I discovered the essay was less about the government's arbitrary standards, and more about the doctor-patient relationship. The authors emphasized the patient's responsibility in his own healthcare, and the doctor's responsibility as well.

Yes, there is a new look for Ferguson, and he is no longer bound by 15 minute office visits. I thank God each day for The Way, The Truth and my new life.

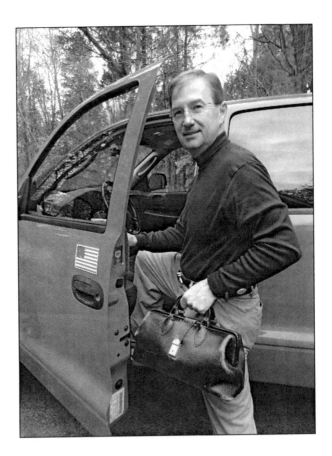

CPSIA information can be obtained at www.ICGtesting.com
Printed in the USA
LVOW07s0737130415

434196LV00005B/8/P